W9-AZR-599

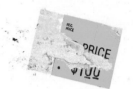

Prisoners
of Psychiatry

Prisoners
of Psychiatry
Mental Patients,
Psychiatrists,
and the Law

Bruce J. Ennis

Introduction by
THOMAS S. SZASZ, M.D.

Harcourt Brace Jovanovich, Inc.
New York

First edition

ISBN 0-15-173084-9

Library of Congress Catalog Card Number: 72-79923

Printed in the United States of America

B C D E

FOR NANCY LEE NORTON

Preface

This is a book about men and women whose lives were changed —and often destroyed—by the label "mental illness." It is also a book about the law, about judges who care and judges who care not at all what happens behind the locked doors of a mental hospital.

There are, right now, nearly three-quarters of a million patients in this nation's mental hospitals. Approximately 400,000 of them reside in state and county mental hospitals, the remainder in V.A. hospitals, private hospitals, and general hospitals with psychiatric wards. Many of them will be physically abused, a few will be raped or killed, but most of them will simply be ignored, left to fend for themselves in the cheerless corridors and barren back wards of the massive steel and concrete warehouses we—but not they—call hospitals. Each day thousands will die (the death rate by age group is much higher in mental hospitals than outside) or be discharged, and other thousands will take their place.

During the coming year, one and a half million Americans will find themselves patients in a mental hospital, most against their wills. At the current admission rate, one out of every ten of us will someday be hospitalized for mental illness; admissions have doubled in the last fifteen years and are steadily rising. Already there are more patients in mental hospitals than in general hospitals, and three times as many mental patients as there are prisoners.

So vast an enterprise will occasionally harbor a sadistic psychiatrist or a brutal attendant, condemned even by his colleagues when discovered. But that is not the central problem. The problem, rather, is the enterprise itself.

The most important function of mental hospitals is to provide custodial welfare. They used to be called insane asylums, but before that they were called, more accurately, poorhouses. Almost all mental patients are poor, or black, or both, and most of them are old.

Less than 5 per cent of those patients are dangerous to themselves or to others. Indeed, the incarceration of mental patients cannot be justified by their threat to the community at large. Studies have shown that they are less dangerous than the "average" citizen. They are put away not because they are, in fact, dangerous, but because they are useless, unproductive, "odd," or "different." We ask psychiatrists to treat them and make them well, but how can we expect psychiatrists to find friends for the friendless, to make the poor rich and the old young? It should not be surprising that they do not even try.

For three years I represented mental patients, trying, as a lawyer, to change the laws that strip them of their liberty and dignity. This is a book about those years.

Contents

Acknowledgments

This book is based upon a litigation project started by the New York Civil Liberties Union, in December of 1968, to protect and expand the rights of mental patients. The project received substantial encouragement and financial support from the NYCLU and its Civil Liberties Defense and Education Fund, the ACLU and its ACLU Foundation, The Norman Foundation, the New York Foundation, the Van Ameringen Foundation, The Carol Buttenwieser Loeb Foundation, and the Ottinger Foundation.

I wish to thank Loren Siegel and Lewis Novod for their assistance during the first half of the project, and Linda Pinckney for her help from that point on. Ira Glasser made valuable suggestions and Robert Christgau deserves special mention for his extensive editorial assistance.

Finally, I wish to thank my clients for permission to use their stories and, in most cases, their real names.

Introduction

I

The coercion and restraint of the mental patient by the psychiatrist is coeval with the origin and development of psychiatry. As an organized discipline, American psychiatry began in the early nineteenth century, with the construction of mental hospitals. In 1844, thirteen superintendents of mental hospitals joined to form the Association of Medical Superintendents of American Institutions for the Insane, the organization that became, in 1921, the American Psychiatric Association.

The original name of this first American psychiatric organization is revealing; and so is its first official resolution. The group's name articulated its character: it was an organization of "medical superintendents," that is, of physicians who were in charge of incarcerated individuals considered and called insane. The organization's first official proposition was: "Resolved, that it is the unanimous sense of this convention that the attempt to abandon entirely the use of all means of personal restraint is not sanctioned by the true interests of the insane."[1]

Ever since, this paternalistic justification of psychiatric coercion has been a prominent theme in psychiatry, not only in America but throughout the civilized world. In 1967—123 years after the drafting of its first resolution—the American Psychiatric Association again reaffirmed its support of psychiatric coercion and restraint. In a "Position Statement on the Question of the Adequacy of Treatment," the association declared that "restraints may be imposed [on the patient] from within by pharmacologic means or by locking the door of a ward. Either imposition may be a legitimate component of a treatment program."[2]

These resolutions must be placed in their proper historical context. In the early days of American psychiatry, alienists justified involuntary psychiatric interventions by appeals to the "true interests of the insane." At the same time, they apparently readily reconciled themselves to the fact that it was not necessary to be, or to be declared, insane to justify incarceration in an insane asylum. In one jurisdiction, it was enough to be a married woman: the 1851 Illinois commitment law states that "married women . . . may be entered or detained in the hospital [the state asylum at Jacksonville, Illinois] at the request of the husband of

1. Quoted in Nina Ridenour, *Mental Health in the United States: A Fifty Year History* (Cambridge: Harvard University Press, 1961), p. 76.
2. Council of the American Psychiatric Association, "Position Statement on the Question of Adequacy of Treatment," *American Journal of Psychiatry*, 123:1458–1460 (May), 1967, p. 1459.

the woman . . . without evidence of insanity required in other cases."[3]

Nowadays, psychiatrists justify involuntary psychiatric interventions by appeals to the requirements of a "legitimate . . . treatment program" for the mentally sick patient. This justification must be viewed in the light of the fact that many psychiatrists are now ready to classify anyone and everyone as mentally sick, and anything and everything as psychiatric treatment.

The result was, and is, an apparently irrefutable justification of psychiatric force and fraud—a justification based on ostensibly altruistic motives and considerations: the "true interests" of the insane, 130 years ago; the "therapeutic needs" of the mental patient, today.

Similar justifications for involuntary psychiatric interventions of all kinds, and especially involuntary mental hospitalization, have, of course, been advanced, and continue to be advanced, in other countries.

In short, just as, for millennia, involuntary servitude has been accepted as a proper economic and social arrangement, so, for centuries, involuntary psychiatry has been accepted as a proper medical and therapeutic arrangement.[4]

II

There are some signs that now point to a shift in this long-established popular and professional position on involuntary mental hospitalization. For example, only ten years ago, St. Elizabeths Hospital, the American government's model mental hos-

3. Quoted in Albert Deutsch, *The Mentally Ill in America: A History of Their Care and Treatment from Colonial Times*, 2nd ed. (New York: Columbia University Press, 1952), p. 424.
4. Thomas S. Szasz, *Ideology and Insanity: Essays on the Psychiatric Dehumanization of Man* (Garden City, N.Y.: Doubleday Anchor, 1970), pp. 113–139.

pital in Washington, D.C., was generally regarded as a fine, "progressive" mental hospital. No one—the best authorities assured us—was confined within its walls who did not belong there. Dr. Winfred Overholser—who was then the superintendent of St. Elizabeths, who had been a president of the American Psychiatric Association, and who was a widely respected, indeed, a revered, psychiatrist—viewed himself, and tried to make others view him, as a protector of the mental patient's civil rights. At the 1961 hearings of the Senate Subcommittee on Constitutional Rights, Dr. Overholser testified that "unfounded fears have been created regarding possible unlawful deprivation of liberty of the patient. . . . After 45 years in mental hospitals and their administration, I am convinced that the basis for the belief that persons are improperly sent to mental hospitals is, for practical purposes, entirely without foundation."[5]

In contrast to this assertion, consider a series of recent articles in the Washington newspapers. In one, titled "Who Really Needs to Be at St. Elizabeths?" we read: "A recent survey at St. Elizabeths Hospital found that 68 per cent of the patients had 'no behavior problem' requiring them to stay in the hospital. Doctors reported that 2,451 inpatients, representing two-thirds of the total, in effect did not have to live in a mental institution. 'None of these patients could be considered dangerous to themselves or others by any definition of the terms,' the report said. . . . The hospital's findings are contained in a confidential preliminary report of a patient inventory conducted by the staff in June, 1970, the first of its kind at St. Elizabeths."[6]

How are we to account for this difference at St. Elizabeths in the decade between 1961 and 1971? Is it that as long as Dr. Over-

5. Winfred Overholser, Statement, in *Constitutional Rights of the Mentally Ill* (Washington, D.C.: U.S. Government Printing Office, 1961), pp. 19–40; p. 21.
6. Robert Pear, "Who Really Needs to Be at St. Elizabeths?" *Washington Evening Star*, August 9, 1971, p. A-1.

holser was alive and at the head of this hospital only those need-
ing confinement were committed, but that since his death, under
the regime of his successors, two out of every three persons were
falsely committed? That is one possibility. I think it's a very remote one.

Another possibility is that the patient population at St. Elizabeths has not changed significantly during the past decade, but
that Dr. Overholser was sincerely mistaken or cravenly mendacious in his judgment of who should and who should not be confined at his hospital. I think this is a more likely explanation.

Of special significance in these reports is the attitude of the
press toward this procedure. Until recently, in exposés of mental
hospitals (of which there was never a shortage), the emphasis
was invariably on the inadequacy of the treatment received by
the "patients." In the press, the idea that the people confined in
mental hospitals were sick and needed treatment was never
questioned. This assumption is apparently no longer held quite
so blindly. For example, an editorial in the *Washington Evening Star* entitled "People Storage" begins as follows: "What
does it take these days to qualify people for lodgment in a mental
institution? For many people, not much in the way of mental
instability."[7]

III
Another sign of a fundamental change in the United States
toward involuntary mental hospitalization, and perhaps the most
important and most hopeful one, is the new position on this
subject by civil libertarians—in particular by members of the
American Civil Liberties Union. One result of this change is the
pioneering project of the New York Civil Liberties Union on
behalf of persons accused of mental illness, reported by Bruce

7. Editorial, "People Storage," *Washington Evening Star*, August 11, 1971.
   p. A-18.

Ennis in his moving chronology of medical abuses committed by psychiatrists under the auspices of the New York State Department of Mental Hygiene and other authorities. To appreciate the full significance of *Prisoners of Psychiatry*, this work, too, must be seen in the context of its historical development.

Until a few years ago, the New York Civil Liberties Union, as well as its parent organization, the American Civil Liberties Union, saw psychiatric problems through the lens formed by the imagery and rhetoric of psychiatry. In this view, what the involuntarily hospitalized mental patient needs is not liberty, but treatment. In its "Position Statement on Involuntary Mental Hospitalization," issued in March, 1972, the American Psychiatric Association reiterated this stand in the following words: "The American Psychiatric Association is convinced that most persons who need hospitalization for mental illness can be and should be informally and voluntarily admitted to hospitals in the same manner that hospitalization is afforded for any other illness. . . . Unfortunately, a small percentage of patients who need hospitalization are unable, because of their mental illness, to make a free and informed decision to hospitalize themselves. Their need for and right to treatment in a hospital cannot be ignored. In addition, public policy demands that some form of involuntary hospitalization be available for those mentally ill patients who constitute a danger either to themselves or to others. In such cases, it is a public responsibility to guarantee the right to treatment. . . ."[8]

The American Civil Liberties Union has long supported this position. In his account of the history of the ACLU, Charles Markmann notes that, toward the end of World War II, "the Union . . . began to draft model statutes for the commitment of the insane. . . . Twenty years after the first Union draft of a

8. American Psychiatric Association, "Position Statement on Involuntary Mental Hospitalization," *American Journal of Psychiatry*, 128:1480 (May), 1972.

model bill for commitments to mental hospitals, Congress enacted for the District of Columbia a law closely following the Union's proposal."[9]

Thus, as recently as 1965, model commitment laws sponsored by the ACLU were hailed with pride by a civil libertarian historian of the Union. Furthermore, although, in 1969, the New York Civil Liberties Union passed a resolution rejecting involuntary mental hospitalization as incompatible with the principles of a free society,[10] the American Civil Liberties Union has, to this date, not followed suit. Its continued support of commitment—now more tacit than explicit—is consistent with the fact that one of the vice-chairmen of its National Committee has been, and continues to be, Karl Menninger, one of the staunchest and most influential psychiatric supporters of involuntary mental hospitalization.

IV

In short, then, *Prisoners of Psychiatry* must be seen as a manifestation of the growing rejection of the viciously mendacious psychiatric rhetoric about "mental illness"; and of the corresponding recognition that individuals incriminated as mentally ill do not need guarantees of "treatment," but protection against their enemies—the legislators, judges, and psychiatrists who persecute them in the name of mental health.

Inasmuch as this frontal attack on the abuses of psychiatry—an attack that seeks to abolish involuntary psychiatric interventions rather than, as did former criticisms, to reform the existing psychiatric institutions—rests, in part, on my critical analyses of psychiatric principles and practices published over the past fif-

9. Charles L. Markmann, *The Noblest Cry: A History of the American Civil Liberties Union* (New York: St. Martin's Press, 1965), pp. 400–401.
10. Resolution of the Board of Directors, January 13, 1969, Minutes, p. 3.

teen years,[11] it may be useful to summarize those of my views that support Mr. Ennis's presentation and conclusions, and are in turn supported by them.

1. The term "mental illness" is a metaphor. More particularly, as this term is used in mental hygiene legislation, "mental illness" is not the name of a medical disease or disorder, but is a quasi-medical label whose purpose is to conceal conflict as illness and to justify coercion as treatment.

2. If "mental illness" is an illness "like any other illness"—as official medical, psychiatric, and mental health organizations, such as the American Medical Association, the American Psychiatric Association, and the National Association for Mental Health, maintain—then it follows, logically and semantically, that it must be treated like any other illness. Hence, mental hygiene laws must be repealed. There are no special laws for patients with peptic ulcer or pneumonia; why, then, should there be special laws for patients with depression or schizophrenia?

3. If, on the other hand, "mental illness" is, as I contend, a metaphor and a myth, then, also, it follows that mental hygiene laws should be repealed.

4. If there were no mental hygiene laws—which alone have the legal power to create a category of individuals who, though officially labeled as "mentally ill," would prefer not to be subjected to involuntary psychiatric interventions—then the misdeeds now committed by those who "care" for "mental patients" could not come into being.

5. In short, all those who draft and administer laws pertaining to involuntary psychiatric interventions should be regarded as the adversaries, not the allies, of the so-called mental patient. Civil

11. See especially Thomas S. Szasz, *The Myth of Mental Illness: Foundations of a Theory of Personal Conduct* (New York: Hoeber-Harper, 1961); *Law, Liberty, and Psychiatry: An Inquiry into the Social Uses of Mental Health Practices* (New York: Macmillan, 1963); and *Psychiatric Justice* (New York: Macmillan, 1965).

libertarians, and, indeed, all men and women who believe that no one should be deprived of liberty except upon conviction for a crime, should oppose all forms of involuntary psychiatric intervention.

V

Although *Prisoners of Psychiatry* is an unsettling book, I hope it will be widely read and seriously thought about. And I particularly hope that Americans in increasing numbers will begin to discriminate between two types of physicians: those who heal, not so much because they are saints, but because *that is their job;* and those who harm, not so much because they are sinners, but because *that is their job.* And if some doctors harm—torture rather than treat, murder the soul rather than minister to the body—that is, in part, because society, the state, asks them, and pays them, to do so.

We saw it happen in Nazi Germany, and we hanged many of the doctors.

We see it happen in the Soviet Union, and we denounce the doctors with righteous indignation.

But when will we see the same things happening in the United States? When will we recognize—and publicly identify—the medical criminals among us? Or is the very possibility of perceiving many of our leading psychiatrists and psychiatric institutions in this way precluded by the fact that they represent the officially "correct" views and practices? By the fact that they have the ears of our legislators and judges? And by the fact that they control the vast funds, collected by the state through taxing the citizens, which finance an enterprise whose basic moral legitimacy is here called into question?

THOMAS S. SZASZ, M.D.

Prisoners
of Psychiatry

Part I
The Criminal
and the King

Mental illness is mental illness, whether it afflicts the criminal or the king.
—THE HONORABLE IRVING R. KAUFMAN
United States Circuit Judge

Most of the patients in mental hospitals are civil patients, people who have not committed any crime or broken any law. There are, however, a few mental hospitals for the "criminally insane." The label is misleading because only a few of the "criminal" patients have been convicted of a crime. Most "criminal" patients are persons who have been accused of crime, but who have not yet been convicted. Instead of being brought to trial, to establish their innocence or guilt, they are judged to be mentally "incompetent" to stand trial and are committed to a mental hospital, where they will remain until, in the opinion of the authorities, they regain competence. Then, and only then, will they have a chance to prove their innocence.

These four chapters are about people who have been labeled criminally insane. The stories are true, and they are not at all unusual. During my three years as director of the New York Civil Liberties Union's Civil Liberties and Mental Illness Litigation Project, I represented dozens of persons in Matteawan and Dannemora, New York's hospitals for the "criminally insane." I include these four stories, rather than others, only because these were the first to reach my attention.

I started working on Jerome Wright's case on my first day at the Civil Liberties Union. Within one month, I was representing Charlie Youngblood and Theodore Neely, Jr., and, a month later, Alfred Curt von Wolfersdorf.

These stories are not the cream of the crop; they are not carefully selected for their shock value from a mass of humdrum cases. If they are disturbing, it is precisely because they are so common.

1 / "No One Keeps a Lion for a Pet"

January 18, 1969, started like any other day, with a telephone call: "Mr. Ennis, my name is Charlie Youngblood. I'm crazy but competent."

"What?"

"I can elucidate and I don't hallucinate."

"What are you talking about?"

"The United States attorney is trying to murder me."

"I don't understand."

"He says I'm not competent to stand trial for a violation of Title 18 United States Code, section 875."

5

"What's that?"

"Communicating in interstate commerce a threat to injure the person of another."

"And you want to stand trial?"

"Yes, I want to stand trial. They don't want to try me because if they did, every man in that courtroom would go to jail for misprision* of a felony in violation of Title 18 United States Code, sections 241 and 242."

"Why does the United States attorney think you are incompetent to stand trial?"

"He knows I'm *competent*—they just don't want to try me. They want to put me in a mental hospital where I'll die."

To Youngblood, competence to stand trial was more important than guilt or innocence. If convicted on the criminal charge of threatening to injure another, he could receive at most a five-year sentence; if found incompetent, he would probably spend the rest of his life in a mental hospital—Youngblood had been diagnosed as a paranoid schizophrenic for twenty-five years, and it was unlikely that his mental condition would improve in the future. The incompetency proceeding was therefore comparable to a prosecution for murder. Before I could agree to represent Youngblood, I needed to know a lot more about his case.

The next day, a Sunday, Charlie Youngblood lumbered into my office right on time, laden with letters, Veterans Administration documents, transcripts of various V.A. hearings, and a tape recorder. He was a big man, particularly in the shoulders. He had a large square face, flat yellowish eyes, a broad flaring nose, and meaty hands the color of creamed coffee. Gesturing aggressively, Youngblood hunched over my desk and told his story.

According to the government, on the morning of October 2, 1968, Youngblood had picked up the telephone in his apartment

---

* "Misprision" means failure to prevent or report a crime.

on Boynton Avenue in the Bronx and called Attorney General Ramsey Clark in Washington, D.C., threatening to "break his ass" if he didn't do something about the Veterans Administration's refusal to rule upon Youngblood's claim for additional service-connected disability benefits. Nor had Youngblood's list stopped with Clark. It had included, said the government, several lawyers in the Justice Department and key men in the New York City office of the V.A. It turned out that Youngblood had been in constant battle with the government for twenty-five years; indeed, fighting the government was his life's work. His troubles had started with a pair of boots.

On December 11, 1943, eighteen-year-old Charlie Youngblood was inducted into the United States Army at Camp Upton, Long Island, where he was issued one pair of army boots, size eleven. No matter that Youngblood wore nines; the camp was out of nines, and he was forced, despite repeated protest, to wear the oversized shoes. After three months of basic training in Gulfport, Mississippi, his feet hurt so much that he threw the boots away and went barefoot until, finally, he was issued the correct size.

As might be expected in the Deep South of that day, Youngblood and the other blacks in training at Gulfport were subject to various harassments. From time to time, Youngblood received letters from his father, Captain Edwin B. Youngblood, one of the highest-ranking blacks in the Army. When the other G.I.s, most of whom were white, got onto this, they began to pester Youngblood—"You think you're better than us because your father's a captain, don't you?"; "Any orders for us today, captain?" Twice, while sleeping, he was pushed from his upper bunk to the concrete floor, only to hear "Sorry about that, captain," from a pack of snickering G.I.s.

At a movie one Saturday night, several soldiers told Youngblood he would have to move to the "colored" section of the theater. More from personal pride than from racial consciousness (he did not think of himself as Negro or colored, but, as he would say again and again in the next twenty-five years, "the one thing I am, above all, is an American"), Youngblood refused to move, pointing out that the colored section—small to begin with—was already overcrowded, while the white section was nearly empty. After an argument, Youngblood stormed out to the ticket window to get his money back, followed by a few of the white G.I.s. When one of them pulled a knife, Youngblood swept the cashbox out through the ticket window, scattering coins and bills onto the sidewalk. It was an old trick, but it worked; enough of his assailants went for the money to enable Youngblood to fight his way free. Late the next day, the base commander accused Youngblood of "provoking an incident" and ordered him, as punishment, to man a remote guard post located on a dirt road at the very edge of the camp. The guard post had been built earlier that day.

As evening came, Youngblood left his post and crouched a few yards away in a shallow ravine. Soon he heard the rumble of an army truck coming over a rise, moving fast in the Mississippi night—too fast for a truck traveling without lights. Veering off the dusty road, the truck crashed through the makeshift guard post, leaving nothing but splinters. Youngblood scrambled out of the ravine, fired once at the receding truck, and fled.

The Army found him ten days later in the chicken coop of an upstate Mississippi farm and sent him under guard to Utah, where, on May 13, 1944, five months after his induction, he received a "Section VIII discharge from the armed forces for undesirable habits and traits of character." He had been "disqualified in character for service, through his own misconduct." The discharge also contained a psychiatric element. According to a V.A. "clinical record" dated January 10, 1961, the "military psychiatrist, in 1944, reported a pattern of acting out, grandiose and inappropriate behavior, hallucinations, and homicidal tendencies."

Immediately upon separation, Youngblood filed a formal request to change his discharge from a Section VIII to a medical discharge. He claimed that as a direct consequence of improper footwear he had incurred flat feet (*pes planus* was the medical term he used), and that the prejudice, harassment, and brutality of life at the Gulfport base had caused whatever mental abnormalities the Army attributed to him.

Prior to induction, no one had thought Youngblood crazy. He had played semiprofessional basketball on the "Eastern" circuit —a night game in Saratoga, then on to Glens Falls, Geneva, Oswego, and back to Chester, Pennsylvania—for $250 a week, an unlikely living for a man with flat feet. Besides, his feet and his mind had passed without question at the preinduction examination.

For those service-connected disabilities Youngblood demanded a medical discharge and financial compensation. He got neither. For the next fifteen years he drifted from one job to another, working on the docks of New York, in the post office, and in construction. He left each job—or was fired—because of a "nervous condition due to military service," as he put it.

On March 27, 1960, Youngblood was in an automobile accident in which his left leg and foot were crushed and his right ankle fractured. He was shunted from one hospital to another —including the psychiatric division of Bellevue for a ten-day stopover—and wound up in the Bronx V.A. Hospital on June 27, three months to the day after his accident. Because he was hard to manage, the staff administered daily injections of chlorpromazine, more commonly known as Thorazine, a tranquilizing medication frequently prescribed for mental patients. After a few days on Thorazine, Youngblood began to feel ill. It seemed to him that the tranquilizer was "poisoning" his system. The authorities paid no attention—Youngblood was, after all, "crazy"—until, on July 20, 1960, they finally ran a test and found "blood chemistries compatible with hepatic [liver] dysfunction." In short, like thousands of other mental patients, Youngblood had become seriously jaundiced from a sensitivity reaction to Thorazine.

His doctors discontinued the medication, set up a round-the-clock personal nursing schedule, and reversed the jaundice. But they did not save his foot. In September, two months after admission and six months after the accident, "the 3rd left toe had undergone spontaneous amputation" (that is, it fell off), and, in October, the "2nd left toe was amputated surgically because of gangrene and resulting osteomyelitis," the result, according to Youngblood, of hospital neglect. His left leg never healed properly. For most of July, August, and September the leg was in a cast, followed by two months in a splint. In early December, Youngblood was sent home for the weekend, though still on crutches. The next day, as he left his apartment, his left leg buckled and he was rehospitalized. This time the hospital put him in a full-body spica cast, where he remained, totally immobile, for more than six months.

In July of 1961, shortly after the cast was removed, Youngblood left the hospital "AMA"—against medical advice—and began a one-man letter-writing campaign to persuade Congress to investigate the "inadequate and unskillful" medical care he had received. Much later, in May of 1970, *Life* reported that a Senate subcommittee headed by California's Alan Cranston had conducted a five-month investigation of V.A. hospitals and had documented "gross inadequacies," particularly in the hospital where Youngblood had spent more than a year of his life. The Bronx V.A. Hospital was described as "more antiquated than most," a "medical slum," and a place "so full of rodents that a trap set on any given evening usually produces a mouse or rat by morning." Paraplegic patients had to wash and dress each other as best they could; therapy was almost nonexistent. Dirty linen accumulated on urine-stained floors; overcrowded patients shared corners with trash cans. It was a dismal picture, and it bolstered Youngblood's contention that he had spent a year on his back and lost two toes because of hospital indifference.

In June of 1964, twenty years after his discharge from the

Army, Youngblood finally got an appellate hearing on his claim for service-connected disability. Taking the train to Washington, D.C., he represented himself before the three-man Board of Veterans Appeals. After setting out fully his claim for psychiatric and *pes planus* benefits, he went on to explain his more recent claim for liver damage and inadequate treatment in the Bronx V.A. Hospital. The hearing was cordial; the panel even seemed somewhat sympathetic to Youngblood's presentation, which was, as always, flamboyant and impassioned. Two weeks later it denied all his claims except the one for psychiatric disability benefits. The panel found that his mental condition—characterized as paranoid schizophrenia—was indeed service connected, thus entitling him to compensation; but, because of a procedural technicality, it refused to make the payments retroactive to the date of his discharge. He was told he would have to undergo psychiatric evaluation to determine the degree of disability; only after he had been evaluated would the first of his monthly checks be forwarded.

Youngblood was not satisfied with the decision, and he intended to appeal, but a small check was better than none, so he signed into the Albany V.A. Hospital for a psychiatric evaluation. There, he was given the same drugs that had nearly killed him in 1960. On December 9, 1964, the day scheduled for his "sanity hearing," nurses came to his ward early in the morning to administer another injection, but he feigned grogginess and they let him alone. A few hours later attendants lifted him into a wheelchair and rolled him to a small amphitheater for what was described as a "psychiatric conference with Dr. Holt presiding." According to the hospital's clinical record, Youngblood "rapidly dominated the interview." He listened with bowed head while a doctor described his mental disability, but when the doctor began to insist that Youngblood was so severely handicapped that he was not even competent to handle his own disability checks, and that all payments should go to a "guardian,"

Youngblood opened his eyes, threw off his blanket, and sprang out of his wheelchair to address the panel:

You thought you were feeding the Christian to the lions when you wheeled me in here, but when you opened the door to let me in this hospital you did not let in a Christian, you let in a lion, and no one keeps a lion for a pet.

In equally colorful language, liberally sprinkled with psychiatric and legal terms, as well as a few obscenities, Youngblood parried the doctors' questions about his financial needs and his ability to handle money, and walked out of the hospital with an allowance of $250 per month. He thought he was entitled to more (six years later, after more battles with the V.A., he would be getting $500 per month, still less than he claimed), but it was the first service-connected check he had received since his discharge twenty years earlier, and he was encouraged to press on.

Although his own claims took up most of his time, Youngblood was fast becoming an expert on V.A. benefits and procedures—so expert, in fact, that he soon began to represent other veterans who had grievances against the V.A. Serving as a lay advocate without compensation, he won more than he lost and recovered a substantial amount of money for his "clients."

From 1964 through 1968, Youngblood repeatedly tried to persuade the V.A. to reconsider his claim for retroactive benefits. He was told that the claim was no longer under V.A. jurisdiction, that his only recourse was to the Justice Department in Washington, D.C. So Youngblood peppered the Justice Department with requests for assistance, and on August 21, 1968, he traveled to Washington to discuss his claim with Morton Sklar and Stuart Nelkin, attorneys in the Justice Department. Finally, on August 27, 1968, Nelkin wrote Youngblood that "the Veterans Administration now acknowledges that your complaints are properly within the scope of its authority rather than within that of the Justice Department." But on August 30, only three days later, Youngblood got a letter from Dan Grody, adjudication officer of the New York office of the V.A., again denying responsibility for Youngblood's claim. Youngblood would not give up. Another letter to Sklar on September 10 brought no response, so on October 2, 1968, certain he would never get action unless he went to the top, Youngblood called the Justice Department and asked to speak to the attorney general, Ramsey Clark.

Youngblood was angry and the secretary who answered the telephone became alarmed. She left the phone for a few seconds and then asked, "Are you threatening the attorney general?"

"You gotta be kidding," he replied; but she would not put the call through, and he hung up. The next day, FBI agents called Youngblood and asked him to come down to their Manhattan office, where he was arrested and charged with threatening to injure Ramsey Clark, Stuart Nelkin, Morton Sklar, and Dan Grody. On the fourth, agents Patrick J. O'Conner, Stuart Senneff, and Robert Fox took Youngblood before Commissioner Earle N. Bishopp, who set bail at $1,000. Three days later, Youngblood managed to raise the bail and was released from jail.

Youngblood was actually looking forward to the criminal trial; he was sure he could prove his innocence, and he hoped to use the courtroom as a forum for airing his complaints about the V.A. But the assistant U.S. attorney in charge of the case, Richard Ben-Veniste, had other ideas; he had begun proceedings to have Youngblood declared incompetent to stand trial. The hearing on his mental condition was set for March 10, 1969. Ben-Veniste had already obtained a court order directing Youngblood to submit to a psychiatric examination by Dr. David Abrahamsen, a private psychiatrist retained by the government. Youngblood didn't trust the government, and he certainly didn't trust a government psychiatrist, so he smuggled in a tape recorder and managed to record more than half the interview before it was discovered.

Also, acting entirely on his own, Youngblood decided he would need expert testimony that he was competent. On January 27, 1969, nine days after he had first called my office, he went to the Soundview-Throgs Neck Community Mental Health Center, a free clinic for residents of the Bronx, and asked to be examined. The first I knew of that was a telephone call from Dr. Jonathan Cohen, a psychiatrist and associate director of the center. There was a man in his office, he said, named Charlie Youngblood, who claimed I was his lawyer. I told him that was true, explained the purpose of the March 10 competency hearing, and asked if he thought Youngblood was competent to stand trial. I smiled at the resourcefulness of my "incompetent" client as I jotted down Dr. Cohen's reply: "I have no doubt at all that this man is competent to stand trial." Dr. Manfred Behrens, a psychiatrist and director of the center, agreed. Youngblood was not going to be sent to a mental hospital without a fight.

My first legal maneuver was to make a motion to postpone the competency hearing until the government had obtained an indictment. The grand jury, which is the only body empowered to indict, had not yet considered whether the complaint against Youngblood warranted a trial. The motion was based on several statutory and constitutional grounds, but underlying them all was the common-sense notion that a defendant's competence to stand trial should not be questioned until the government has established the probability of a trial for which he need be competent. For a felony, that requires a grand jury indictment. If the court were to commit Youngblood to a mental hospital, and if the government thereafter proved unable to obtain an indictment, he would have been unnecessarily deprived of liberty. The court denied my motion, but in doing so it specifically adopted a major premise of the motion, that the government would have to get an indictment *sometime,* either before the competency hearing or, at the least, "promptly" after an order of commitment.

The Southern District of New York (which includes Manhattan) thus joined the Western District of Missouri as the only judicial districts in the entire federal system that expressly recognize that a defendant cannot constitutionally be permitted to languish forever in a mental hospital if the probability of his being brought to trial rests on nothing more substantial than a complaint. That ruling will help other defendants—it will protect them from frivolous complaints filed by hostile neighbors, for example—but it did not help Youngblood. Within the month Ben-Veniste sought and obtained a grand jury indictment.

My next step was to demand a jury trial on the issue of Youngblood's competence. Even though a finding of incompetency frequently results in a longer period of incarceration than a finding of guilt, it is an almost invariable rule throughout the United States that allegedly incompetent defendants are not entitled to the protection of a jury trial. My motion was based upon the Sixth Amendment to the United States Constitution, which guarantees that in "all criminal prosecutions" the accused shall enjoy the right to trial "by an impartial jury," and upon another provision of the Constitution (Article III, Section 2, Clause 3), which states unequivocally that "the Trial of all Crimes, except in Cases of Impeachment, shall be by Jury." In a 1942 case, the United States Supreme Court had ruled that the object of the latter provision "was to preserve unimpaired trial by jury in all those cases in which it had been recognized by the common law." By the common law, the Court meant the body of law that had developed in the English courts prior to the adoption of the Constitution.

I spent a week reading dusty volumes in the basement of the

New York University Law School Library and discovered, to my surprise, that at common law the issue of competence to stand trial *was* tried by jury. In his *Commentaries*, Lord Blackstone (described by the Supreme Court as the "most satisfactory expositor" of the common law) put it this way: "If there be any doubt, whether the party be compos [competent to stand trial] or not, this shall be tried by a jury." From my reading of the *Frith* case, *Rex* v. *Pritchard*, and many other eighteenth-century English authorities, it was clear to me that at common law only a jury could finally declare a defendant incompetent to stand trial.

Nevertheless, the court denied my motion for a jury trial, pointing out that the incompetency proceeding is, at least technically, a civil proceeding, not a criminal proceeding. Accordingly, present-day defendants cannot demand the jury trial to which their forefathers were entitled under the common law. Equally important, labeling the incompetency proceeding civil rather than criminal means that the government has to prove the defendant incompetent not "beyond a reasonable doubt" (the criminal standard), but only by a "preponderance of the evidence" (the civil standard). Under the civil standard, a defendant can be found incompetent if the government's evidence of incompetence is only slightly more persuasive than the defendant's evidence of competence. Under the criminal standard, a defendant can be found incompetent only if the evidence of incompetence is overwhelmingly stronger than the evidence of competence. The use of the civil standard thus makes it a lot easier for the government to commit defendants to mental hospitals against their will.

Unlike most competency trials, which are rather perfunctory (hearings of two or three minutes are not uncommon), Youngblood's trial lasted two days. I knew I could not persuade Judge Charles M. Metzner that Youngblood was entirely sane—even our own psychiatrists thought he was a paranoid schizophrenic

—but I hoped to persuade him that a defendant can be severely ill in psychiatric terms and still be *legally* competent to stand trial. In order to make the issue as precise as possible, I hoped Dr. Abrahamsen, the government's psychiatrist, would say that *anyone* diagnosed as a paranoid schizophrenic should *automatically* be considered incompetent to stand trial; I knew that my witnesses, Doctors Cohen and Behrens, would disagree.

Abrahamsen testified first, stressing that during the psychiatric interview Youngblood had said, "You are going to murder me for $75," the amount the court had previously set as Abrahamsen's fee (he ultimately got $150). Abrahamsen repeated that statement nine times during his testimony, and seven times he referred to Youngblood's statement that "people have tried to murder me through poisoning." That, said Abrahamsen, proved Youngblood was paranoid and incompetent to stand trial.

I began my cross-examination by asking if Youngblood had ever explained what he meant when he said that Abrahamsen was going to murder him for $75.

A. No, he did not explain anything. He only said that "you are going to murder me for $75," and I don't believe that needs any explanation.
Q. He never qualified in any respect what he meant by the word "murder"?
A. No.
Q. You are certain of that?
A. Absolutely.

I left that point for the moment and asked if Youngblood had explained what he meant when he said "people have tried to murder me through poisoning." "No," said Abrahamsen, "I tried to get an explanation of it, but he could not elaborate on it." Within two minutes, however, Abrahamsen admitted that Youngblood had showed him V.A. records that described the jaundice and hepatitis he had suffered as a sensitivity reaction to Thorazine.

Q. Then I will ask you again if he made any explanation of what he meant when he said that he was going to be poisoned?

A. Yes. This condition about hepatitis came about because of the medication he was given.

After a little more skirmishing, Abrahamsen finally admitted that it would be "reasonable for the defendant to believe that were he hospitalized and given this medication, it would poison his system, in fact." Abrahamsen had as much as conceded that one of his specific examples of Youngblood's incompetence—fear of poisoning—was far from conclusive. Hoping he was now ready to fall back on generalities, I asked him casually whether in his opinion "a person" who had been diagnosed as a paranoid schizophrenic would be "competent or incompetent to stand trial."

Ben-Veniste saw what I was doing and jumped to his feet to object. There was nothing improper about the question and he knew it, but he wanted to warn Abrahamsen to be careful. The judge overruled the objection and Abrahamsen, apparently unaware of what Ben-Veniste was trying to tell him, replied, "I believe he would be incompetent to stand trial." The judge, having read my pretrial memorandum of law, knew I was going to argue that a defendant can be severely mentally ill and still be competent to stand trial, and he asked the next question:

Q. All right. Now, anyone who is found to suffer from that mental condition is in your opinion, I understand, mentally incompetent to stand trial?

A. I would be inclined to believe that, sir.

Later, I would show that weeks before Abrahamsen examined Youngblood, he had learned from telephone conversations with

Ben-Veniste and from reading V.A. records that he was a paranoid schizophrenic. The implication was clear—he knew Youngblood was incompetent to stand trial long before he examined
him.

It was time, now, to use the tape of the Abrahamsen-Young-
blood interview, which Youngblood, the paranoid, had so wisely
recorded. The judge would not allow the tape itself to be introduced into evidence, but he did permit me to read from a
typewritten transcript of the tape while questioning Abrahamsen.

At the beginning of the interview Youngblood had told
Abrahamsen that the Civil Liberties Union had agreed to represent him "because there are people being accused of false
crimes and they [the government] use the guise of a psychiatric examination to get rid of them rather than hear the charges.
It is a violation of constitutional law." Then Youngblood had
carefully explained his interpretation of Abrahamsen's role in
the government's case.

YOUNGBLOOD: They're afraid to [prosecute] me. They don't have any
    evidence. And now they want you to find me incompetent so that
    they can throw it out.
ABRAHAMSEN: You don't want it thrown out?
YOUNGBLOOD: No! I want them to bring it out in court.

Youngblood had then explained to Abrahamsen that if he
lost the criminal proceeding, he would at least receive a fixed,
definite sentence; but if Abrahamsen convinced the court that
Youngblood was incompetent, he could "be committed without any definite time period, forever. This is to me murder."
After listening to my quotation from the transcript, Abrahamsen
admitted "that such a matter was discussed." I then pointed out
that Youngblood had explained "that what he meant by 'murder,' when he said you were going to murder him for $75, was to
commit him to a hospital with an indefinite time period." Abra-

hamsen conceded that "it might very well have been so," contradicting his earlier testimony.

Returning to the transcript, I established that Youngblood had told Abrahamsen again and again that "too many people have been put in hospitals, who have been accused of bogus crimes." He was innocent and he wanted the chance to prove it, a chance he would not get if found incompetent and whisked off to a mental hospital. Confronted with the transcript, Abrahamsen's tone changed considerably; he volunteered, for example, that "the outstanding thing I remember was that he was trying to be helpful to people"—an observation he had not included in his written report or in his testimony to that point. Then he admitted, as he had previously denied, that Youngblood "might very well have said" (as in fact he had) that he was "not a murderer" and that he had "no desire to harm people."

Abrahamsen was excused, and Ben-Veniste called John D. Norton of the V.A., who testified that in November of 1966, after he had denied Youngblood's application for training benefits and schooling, Youngblood called on the telephone and threatened "to blow my brains out." On cross-examination Norton conceded that he had not been sufficiently worried to call the police, that Youngblood did not actually do anything, and that there had been no further threats. But the testimony was damaging, and a whole stable of V.A. witnesses waited in the wings to augment it.

Next came Robert Umans, a V.A. dentist. Later, Youngblood would testify that "they took my teeth out in the hospital because of serum and infectious hepatitis. . . . It wasn't until 1966 [five years later] that I was granted teeth. I was allowed to go around with my mouth like it is [removing his false teeth and showing them to the judge] so that I would get a complex from it, an inferiority complex."

But Umans wasn't there to tell that side of the story. I knew from V.A. records that on May 17, 1965, after learning that the

V.A. would not comply with his requests "regarding dental treatment," Youngblood had allegedly called Umans to say that "unless he received his dental treatment, he would come into the office with a knife and cut up everybody that he sees around. If this wasn't effective, he would come in with a hatchet and chop everybody with this razorlike instrument."

Ben-Veniste asked Umans if he recalled speaking on the telephone to a man "who identified himself as Charlie Youngblood." The phrasing of the question stirred a memory from my law-school evidence class, and before Umans could reply, I objected "unless there is previous testimony that he knew the defendant." The point was simple: anyone could call Umans and claim to be Charlie Youngblood. The same objection had occurred to the judge, and when he learned that Umans had met Youngblood only once (after the call) and could not be positive that the person who called and the person he met were one and the same, he sustained the objection. Umans, having nothing further to say, was excused. Ben-Veniste, realizing that the same objection would preclude testimony from his remaining witnesses, announced that "the government has no further witnesses," thus resting the government's case. It was our turn.

During the lunch recess, I realized that Youngblood was absolutely right—the government had no case against him. The October 2 telephone call to the attorney general was the first and last time he had called that office. The secretary who had answered the telephone could not possibly be sure that the caller had been Charlie Youngblood. Even if Youngblood had threatened the attorney general, which he denied, the secretary's testimony would be excluded; and the government had no other evidence. The only hurdle was the incompetency proceeding, which, given Abrahamsen's concessions, we now stood a good chance of winning. But the ever-unpredictable Youngblood, unknown to me, had severely weakened his case by writing a letter to Judge Metzner (to compound matters, the judge had received and read it during the lunch break) in which Youngblood claimed that "your attorney, Richard Ben-Veniste, is conspiring to murder me."

I had known that Youngblood was despondent. He had come to court that morning in old, almost shabby clothes—quite a contrast to his usual caramel-colored leather coat and wing-tipped shoes—and he had left his car and all but one dime at home. So certain was he that he would lose and be sent away for life that he had instructed his wife of two months to give his good clothes and billfold to someone who needed them. But he had not told me about the letter. Before the afternoon session began, the judge, obviously troubled, called me to the bench and showed me the letter, which he marked in evidence as "Court's Exhibit 1."

We called four witnesses, chief among them Doctors Cohen and Behrens, both of whom thought Youngblood was schizophrenic but quite competent to stand trial. As they pointed out, schizophrenia is such an all-inclusive term and covers such a "large range of behavior" that there are few people who could not, at one time or another, be considered schizophrenic. Behrens, for example, said he was then treating on an outpatient basis a doctor and a lawyer, both of whom were, in medical terms, "schizophrenic, paranoid type," but who were continuing to practice their professions and doing "excellent work." It was more important, thought Cohen and Behrens, that Youngblood knew what he was alleged to have done and had been able to provide his attorney with a wealth of material. In fact, it was precisely because he *was* paranoid that he had saved each and every scrap of paper that might be helpful to his case. His memory for names, dates, and places was staggering, far better than the "average" man's. He could certainly provide his attorney with the facts, even though he might exaggerate or misinterpret their significance; from them the attorney could then draw his own conclusions.

Youngblood put aside his crutches and limped to the witness

stand, where he answered my questions in his characteristically precise and concrete manner. "Mr. Youngblood, could you tell the court briefly where you are?"

"Yes, sir. I am in the Federal Court House at Foley Square, zip code 10007."

I asked Youngblood why he had thought it necessary to enlist the aid of Doctors Cohen and Behrens.

Because it is a fact, it is a known fact that this is a conspiracy to murder me, and as I use the term "murder," I plainly stated it, and I have stated it over and over again, it is in telegrams, it is in letters, I have said it over the phone, I have never denied it. Ever since 1960 on, I have said that the Veterans Administration and everyone involved has entered into collusion and conspiracy to murder me, and my definition of that murder is this: I was born free and I will die free. If you take from me my freedom, you have taken from me my life. And to me life is freedom, and other than that, it is murder.

After summarizing his battles with the V.A., including, for example, his four-year struggle to get a special shoe for his crippled left foot, Youngblood pointed out that "I have never once in all these years raised my hand to anyone. I have used the law. And I have corrected these wrongs, a lot of these wrongs."

Ben-Veniste, in cross-examination, asked Youngblood if it wasn't true, however, that he had threatened "to kill" V.A. officials.

With the law. That's my method, that's my gun, the law. The Constitution is my bible. I live and die by the Constitution of the United States because I am an American, that's all I am.

With those words, the hearing closed.

It would be several days before Judge Metzner reached a decision, but late that night Youngblood called me to express his appreciation. "Mr. Ennis, I didn't trust you the first day of the hearings. I didn't trust you the second day, either. I didn't trust you until the end of your closing argument. But I trust you now, and I want you to know that you're the first white man I've trusted in twenty years."

Judge Metzner found that Youngblood was, indeed, a paranoid schizophrenic; but he expressly rejected Dr. Abrahamsen's opinion "that all paranoid schizophrenics are not mentally competent to stand trial." Instead, he ruled—for the first time in any New York federal court—that "such condition does not automatically require a finding of incompetency."

So Youngblood was competent to stand trial. But that did not end his troubles. The V.A. argued that if Youngblood was competent to stand trial there was no reason for him to receive psychiatric disability benefits, and threatened to cut off his monthly checks (it did withhold one) unless he agreed to still another psychiatric examination. And Ben-Veniste asked the court to raise Youngblood's bail to $5,000, a sum he could not meet. Youngblood, on his own, got an order from Judge Walter Mansfield resolving his current difficulties with the V.A., and I got an order from Judge Inzer B. Wyatt reducing Youngblood's bail to zero. That left only the criminal trial.

Twice Youngblood appeared for a "calendar call" and twice the government said it was not ready to go to trial. Finally, in April, 1971, two years after Youngblood had been found competent to stand trial, the government conceded that it had no case and dropped the charges.

2 / Scapegoat

Edward Orman usually drove to work in Manhattan from his new home in Far Rockaway, where he lived with his wife, Eleanor, and their two small children. On December 22, 1966, however, Mrs. Orman needed the car to finish moving. That day, Orman rode the IND subway to the Fulton-Nassau Street stop, got off, and walked toward the staircase connection with the IRT, which would take him on the last leg of his journey. As Orman picked his way through the crowd of clerks and secretaries, a man walking behind him drew a pistol from a paper bag, fired once at Orman's back, and fled down adjoining stairs in time to squeeze through the closing doors on a northbound train. He left Orman crippled for life, with a bullet in his spine. Minutes later, at 8:05 a.m., the police teletype clicked out a description of the assailant: "Male, Negro, 30 years old, 5'8", 150 lbs., slim build, light complexion." No one answering that description would be arrested that day, or the next, or any day thereafter. Thirty-four hours later, a token seller was shot through the left eye at the Fourteenth Street station of the Sixth Avenue subway line, and soon died. Police captured two of his three teen-age assailants; a third remained at large, as did the man who shot Orman.

Many New Yorkers were afraid to ride the subways that Christmas, and the police, aware of the outcry, intensified their investigation; but they had no hard evidence and very few clues—almost nothing to go on.

No one, including Orman, had seen his assailant clearly. But in his haste the man had left something—the police never disclosed what—that led them to believe he was "afraid of germs." Armed with that information and the belief that no one but a madman could commit such a senseless crime, Emile A. Liberatore, of the Old Slip detective squad, one of the city's finest investigative units, sent out queries to all state hospitals, parole officers, clinics, and other institutions that treat mental patients.

Dragnet investigations of mental patients are all too common. Deeply rooted in every society is the erroneous belief that the mentally ill, as a class, are much more dangerous than the mentally healthy. We fear what we do not understand, and it is difficult to understand irrational or unconventional behavior. Not knowing what to expect next from a mental patient, we play it safe and expect the worst. And we are almost always wrong.

The myth that mental patients are more dangerous than the average member of society is not based on empirical evidence, so it is not likely to be destroyed by empirical evidence. The evidence is there, nonetheless. A New York study of 5,000 released mental patients reported that those with no prior criminal record committed less than one-twelfth as many crimes as were committed by "average" members of society; the rate for serious crimes was lower still. Even those patients who did have prior criminal records (most mental patients do not) committed fewer crimes after release than persons with similar criminal records who had not been mental patients. Other studies have reached comparable conclusions.

Lieutenant Liberatore did not look at it that way. Liberatore was a cop, and cops know that between 50 and 80 per cent of all ex-felons will commit additional crimes. They also know that ghetto residents and teen-age males are more likely to commit dangerous acts than the average citizen. But Liberatore did not begin a dragnet investigation of ex-felons, or ghetto residents, or teen-age males. Instead, he concentrated on mental patients, even though they, as a class, are less dangerous than the other three. The Orman shooting had aroused too much public indignation to go unsolved. An arrest would have to be made, and it was becoming more and more likely that the defendant, by a process of elimination, would be a mental patient.

On January 19, 1967, almost a month after Orman's crippling, Lieutenant Liberatore and Detectives Wilbur Oberg and Edward O'Brien drove the fifty miles from Manhattan to Central Islip State Hospital, on Long Island. Central Islip was more like a city than a hospital. It had its own laundry, bakery, and post office. Its 186 buildings on 827 acres of land housed nearly 4,000 employees and more than 8,000 patients. One of those patients was Theodore Neely, Jr. He had been hospitalized a long time—more than seventeen years—and the police had come to arrest him.

The arrest was big news. The *Daily News* for January 20, 1967, carried a picture of Neely under the headline NAB SUBWAY GUN SUSPECT; TRACED BY FEAR OF GERMS. The New York *Times* carried a briefer story under the headline MENTAL PATIENT ON PASS SEIZED IN SUBWAY SHOOTING.

Gwendolyn Lynch, Neely's sister, was puzzled by the newspaper accounts of the assailant's fear of germs because, according to her, Neely was not at all afraid of germs, as his hospital records would show. On the other hand, he did have an aversion to subways and never went near them alone.

The evidence against Neely was entirely circumstantial: he had been in New York City on a holiday pass at the time of the Orman shooting, and he, like the assailant, owned a "salt-and-pepper"-checked sports coat. The police searched the room Neely's parents kept for him in their home in Harlem and found a number of newspapers, including two which described the subway shootings. They did not find the pistol, or any other hard evidence. On February 2, 1967, Neely was indicted by the New York County grand jury, charged with assault in the first degree and related crimes. On July 6, he was found incompetent to stand trial and was committed to Matteawan State Hospital for the criminally insane, to be held there until he became competent. Eleanor Orman accurately mirrored public sentiment when she remarked bitterly that the state would pay for Neely's hospital bill but not for her husband's.

Two years went by, and the public forgot about Theodore Neely and the subway shootings. But Neely's family remembered. On January 14, 1969, Mrs. Willie Mae Neely called me for help. Her son was innocent, she said. Three relatives would swear that at the time of the Orman shooting Neely had been at home, at 460 West 149th Street in Harlem, almost ten miles from the scene of the crime. Two weeks later, at my request, Neely's parents and sister came to my office to fill in the details. I learned then that Teddy, as they called him, did not at all fit the police description of the assailant. He was not five feet, eight inches tall, but almost six feet; not 150 pounds and of slim build, but 200 pounds and powerfully built; not thirty years old, but forty; and, far from having a "light complexion," he was strikingly black, like his sister, Gwendolyn.

Teddy was no ordinary child. He had entered junior high school at the age of nine, three years ahead of playmates his own age, and could have become the youngest high-school graduate in New York City history. But his emotional and social development had not kept pace with his intellectual superiority, and he was removed from school for a time. Hoping that a quieter environment would soften the aggressive spirit that had gotten him in trouble at school, his parents sent Teddy to live with his grandmother in Charlotte, North Carolina, where he finished high school. He even attended college for three years, at Johnson C. Smith University, and planned to enter St. John's Law School.

Neely was a basketball star on his college team until he suffered a head collision with an opposing player, which necessitated a major operation. Shortly thereafter he left college.

According to his parents, Neely was never violent, but his moods changed rapidly from outgoing and talkative to extremely withdrawn and quiet. In early 1950, alarmed by Neely's unstable emotional condition, his parents contacted a private psychiatrist, who visited Neely three times at their home. Neely resented the visits, claiming that the psychiatrist "asked too many foolish questions." Evidently, the psychiatrist recommended that Neely be committed to Central Islip, and his parents reluctantly agreed.

Two years passed and Neely did not improve. Two doctors at Central Islip told Neely's parents that surgery would stabilize Neely's emotions, so they authorized the hospital surgeon to perform a bilateral prefrontal lobotomy, an operation to sever neural connections in the frontal lobe of his brain.

As Professor Phillip Polatin notes in his *Guide to Treatment in Psychiatry*, lobotomy, which was widely "considered a magic remedy" as late as the forties and early fifties, is almost unheard of today, having joined the psychiatric scrap heap of treatments tried and abandoned. In *Lunacy, Law and Conscience*, Kathleen Jones reminds us that the "treatments" rendered to mental patients until the middle of the nineteenth century included repeated dunking in water followed by church services; evacuating the "bad humors" through purges and forced vomiting; bloodletting and the raising of blisters through the application of plasters and hot irons; and, as the historical antecedent of lobotomy, trepanning—boring holes in the patient's skull to allow the bad humors to escape. No doubt the hospital would say the lobotomy "worked" for Teddy; it calmed him down and made him manageable. The second twenty years of his life were not nearly as varied as the first; they proved to be more predictable and so much less eventful that in time he became a "voluntary" patient and later an "honor" patient, free (within limits) to come and go as he chose. It was during one of those leaves that Edward Orman was shot.

After Neely's arrest, the police and, later, a Bellevue psychiatrist questioned him repeatedly. The police offered to reduce the charges and request a suspended sentence if Neely would sign a confession, but throughout the interrogation he insisted he was innocent and wanted to stand trial. Instead, he was shipped off to Matteawan.

Perhaps the lobotomy really had rendered Neely incompetent to stand trial. But what if he was innocent, as he so stoutly claimed? Should he spend the rest of his life in a hospital for the criminally insane simply because he was incompetent to prove his innocence?

In February of 1969, I made the first of three trips to Matteawan to visit Neely. I had never met a lobotomized man, and I didn't know what to expect. Perhaps we would be unable to communicate; worse yet, perhaps my embarrassment would show.

The guard in the gatehouse jotted down my name, the license number of my car, and the purpose of my visit. After noting the hour and minute of my arrival, he let me through the eight-foot cyclone fence, whose presence reminded me that this was not a civil hospital run by the Department of Mental Hygiene, but a hospital for the criminally insane run by the Department of Corrections. I walked the forty or so steps to the ancient T-shaped administration building, paused at the screen door, and entered at the left arm of the T, which houses administrative offices. Down the creaking wooden floors of the other arm, and past the graying 1890's pictures that line the halls—pictures like *The Sitting Room, The Female Dining Room,* or *The Dance of Bacchus* —are the mail-censoring room (another reminder that Matteawan is not like Central Islip) and the financial office. At the neck of the T a display case houses patients' crafts, always the same— porcelain cats, billfolds, and water colors—and behind the case looms an ancient grandfather clock. The clock is silent. Long ago its decorated face came loose and slid to rest askew in the wooden base. It has not been repaired in the three years I have been visiting Matteawan. Perhaps no one has noticed.

One of the ever-present guards told me Neely was "ready" and took me down the shaft of the T to the guardroom, where, again, I signed my name and stated my purpose, noticing as I did so the fingerprint smudges in the visitors' book—at Matteawan, all visitors other than lawyers and doctors, and perhaps clergymen, must be fingerprinted. A guard opened a sliding metal door encrusted with green paint, and we entered a foyer, where two or three more guards stood near a bulletin board passing the time. We turned left down another corridor, this one lined with old school desk-chairs. Three patients, with yet another guard beside them, sat there quietly and followed me with their eyes. At the end of the hall, my escort and I entered the rectangular lunchroom, equipped with long bare tables running its entire length, a few vending machines, and another guard sitting at one end in an elevated, high-backed wooden chair. My escort left me at a table and returned with Neely—one of the three patients I had seen in the hall—who was not permitted to sit next to me, but had to keep his distance across the table. I introduced myself and asked Neely if he had heard anything about me from his family.

"Yes, they were here last weekend and they told me about you."

He had paused before answering, and his words were slow and

deliberate—almost as if he were drugged—but to the point. I was relieved. "Did they tell you what we hoped to do?"

"Yes, they said you would try to get me out of Matteawan and back into a civil hospital."

"Would you rather be in a civil hospital?"

"Yes."

"Why?"

"Well, I would have more freedom—grounds privileges. When I was at Central Islip I worked at the post office."

"You mean you worked there during the day and returned to Central Islip at night?"

"Yes."

His answers were brief, without elaboration, and he had not yet volunteered any information or initiated any questions. Perhaps he was just being polite. I asked if he had any questions.

"Yes. How is the man they say I shot?"

It was obvious that his family had avoided this subject. "He is alive, but paralyzed from the waist down."

Neely frowned. He had pronounced features—deep, wide-set eyes, and a strong, almost square chin. He seem puzzled. "I am sorry about that man," he said slowly, "but I would like to get out of here. I am very sorry for that man and his family, but I don't think I should be punished for that—I don't even know him."

I explained to Neely the principle I hoped to establish in his case. A court had found him to be incompetent to stand trial and had ordered him to remain in Matteawan until he regained competence. Then the state could bring him to trial for the shooting. But since he was unlikely to regain competence, he was in all probability condemned to Matteawan for life. I thought we had enough information to persuade a court to dismiss the indictment against Neely so that he could be transferred back to a civil hospital. There was just one problem. If Neely were competent, he could make a motion to dismiss his indictment for insufficient evidence. However, incompetent defendants did not have that right. Under the law as it then stood, incompetent defendants could not make such motions unless the district attorney consented, which he rarely did. I asked Neely if he followed me so far.

"Yes, I think so."

"Well, I think that law is terrible. It means the D.A. has an absolute veto power, even if you are accusing the D.A. of wrongdoing—withholding relevant information from the grand jury, for example. So before we can move to dismiss the indictment in your case, we must persuade a judge that you have the right to make such a motion whether the D.A. consents or not. I think we can win on that issue, but I don't want to mislead you or get your hopes too high. In order to win we must break new ground. We will have to persuade a judge to do something no judge has ever done before. And that's not easy. So it's up to you. Do you want to try or not?"

"Yes. I don't think I should be held here because of something I didn't do"—it was his first expression of innocence—"and I would like you to do whatever you can."

I took out my billfold and gave Neely a business card, but the guard, who had been hovering twenty feet away, intercepted it and told me he would have to clear it with the director before he could give it to Neely. I asked the guard to do what he could. Then he gave me a three-by-five-inch card on which, once again, I signed my name and stated the purpose of my visit. This time I was asked to add the exact hour and minute at which my interview with Neely had begun and ended. Strange, I thought, thinking of the broken clock in the corridor.

Almost nine months went by. I was working on other cases, and at the same time putting together a lengthy test-case brief for Neely. Then something totally unexpected happened. Every week it was my custom to read through all the latest "advance sheets," weekly pamphlets that report court decisions before they are published in the regular case reports. Skimming through the index one day, I came across *Orman* v. *State of New York*, decided by the New York Court of Claims several months earlier— in fact, on February 18, 1969, the same day I had visited Neely. Could this Orman be the same man Neely was accused of shooting? Racing through the opinion, I froze at the next-to-last paragraph: "It has not been established to the court's satisfaction that the suspect was, in fact, the perpetrator of the assault. . . ."

Edward Orman had sued the State of New York for $1 million, claiming, first, that Neely had shot him, and, second, that the officials at Central Islip had been "negligent" in releasing Neely on a holiday pass, thereby "causing" Orman's injuries. Orman had subpoenaed the police files and introduced "testimony by the police assigned to the criminal case" against Neely. He had also called a witness to the shooting who had testified that he was "reasonably sure but not positive" that Neely was the assailant. In other words, Orman had been able to use almost all the evidence the state would have if it ever brought Neely to trial. But the evidence had not been enough. Although the judge expressed "deep sympathy and concern" for Orman, he noted that "no positive identification was made of the assailant by the Claimant [Orman] nor the witness who heard the shot and saw the flash from it." The judge recognized that Orman's claim against the state did not require proof beyond a reasonable doubt (the criminal standard), but only a preponderance, or majority, of the evidence (the civil standard). Even so, the state was not liable, "since the proof does not warrant the court to hold that the patient on leave [Neely] was the assailant." (Over two years later, a higher court would affirm that decision, though placing more emphasis on the hospital's freedom from negligence than on Neely's innocence.)

We could not have a stronger case. If, using the state's evidence, Orman could not prove in a civil case that Neely was his assailant by a "preponderance of the evidence," how could the state prove Neely's guilt "beyond a reasonable doubt"? The injustice of holding Neely in Matteawan for the rest of his life when he was probably innocent of the criminal charge might prompt a judge to rule unconstitutional the statute that prohibited Neely and other incompetent defendants from challenging their indictments. But not every judge would be willing to go that far. We had to find the right one.

In 1968, a committee of the Association of the Bar of the City of New York had noted with chagrin that there was no statutory "provision authorizing the court to entertain a well-founded motion by counsel challenging the sufficiency of the indictment" against an incompetent defendant, because such "motions require the express consent of the district attorney," which is rarely, if ever, given. The committee thought that "only those aspects of the proceedings requiring the participation of the defendant should be postponed. Counsel should be permitted to make pretrial motions otherwise available to the defendant and, in the circumstances, not requiring his assistance."

One of the members of that Bar Association committee was Jacob Markowitz, a justice of the New York supreme court. (In New York, unlike most states, the supreme court is really the lowest court of general jurisdiction; the highest is the Court of Appeals.) I found out that Judge Markowitz would be sitting for one week, beginning February 2, 1970, in what is called Special Term Part I, the room in the courthouse where Neely's case would have to be argued. Waiting for Judge Markowitz would mean a three-month delay, but considering that there are, in all, nearly seventy-five separate "parts" to which he might have been assigned before Part I, the delay could have been much longer.

Now began the tedious and intricate process of "judge shopping"—an essential skill that is not taught, or even mentioned, in law school. In state-court practice, at least in New York City, it is rare indeed for a motion, a formal request for a court order, to be filed and argued before the first available judge. Lawyers can be reasonably sure of at least one adjournment, and usually more, before their motions are heard. Even if the other side objects, it is not hard to get an adjournment. Each day the "motion calendar" lists about two hundred motions to be heard. One judge simply cannot hear all those motions, not in six hours, not in sixty. Everyone knows that all but a handful of those motions will be "adjourned for a week," dumped in the lap of the next judge, who, in turn, will embrace almost any reason for routing the motion to another of his beleaguered brethren. With new judges coming in each week, it is relatively easy to avoid one you do not want, although hard (without the other side's consent) to hold on to one you do. I wanted Judge Markowitz, and I set out to get him.

The first step was to create an issue, a "justiciable controversy." In a letter to Frank S. Hogan, district attorney for New York County, I reviewed Neely's case and the Orman decision, and requested:

(1) That you consent to dismissal of the indictment, which will make it possible for Neely to be transferred back to Central Islip; or

(2) That you consent to the making of a motion to dismiss the indictment.

Soon came the reply:

After a careful study and evaluation of our file and a discussion of the case with the Assistant District Attorney who presented it to the Grand Jury, this office sees no basis for dismissing the indictment against Mr. Neely.

There is other evidence than that which was apparently presented before the Court of Claims.

Other evidence—what could it be? Well, it might not be so easy to win as I had thought, but at least we had an issue: the

constitutionality of allowing D.A.'s to exercise veto power over
motions made by incompetent defendants.

In early December, I filed a "summons and complaint" challenging the constitutionality of the statute that gave D.A.s this
veto power. The state now had twenty days within which it must
either file an "answer" admitting or denying the factual allegations of the complaint, or must make a "motion to dismiss" the
complaint. On December 29, the state made a motion to dismiss,
which was scheduled to be argued in Special Term Part I on
January 16, 1970—three weeks before Judge Markowitz would be
sitting. Shortly before January 16, I called the assistant district
attorney who was handling the case for the state and told him I
needed an adjournment "for a week or two, or maybe three if
that would be better for you." Three, of course, was what I
wanted—that was "Markowitz week." He suggested Tuesday,
February 3, 1970—fine with me! In order to clinch the date and
forestall a subsequent adjournment, I asked him, pretending not
to know, "Do you know who will be sitting that day?"

"No, I don't."

"Well, that's all right. February 3 will be O.K. with me."

I arrived in the courtroom early. Several lawyers were milling
around shouting out case names in an effort to identify the lawyer
for the other side. I joined them and soon was face to face with
the assistant D.A. We chatted for a few minutes. He was person-
able, reserved, straightforward, even sympathetic to Neely's
plight, though he meant to do all he could to prolong it. Finally
I asked him, "What is this other evidence you have against
Neely?"

He thought for a moment, undecided whether to tell me or
not, and then replied, "Well, when we sent him to Bellevue to
see if he was competent to stand trial, about the only thing he
would say to the psychiatrist was 'They haven't got the gun.
They haven't got the gun.' He kept repeating that over and
over."

"Is that it? Is that your other evidence?"

"Yes," he replied sheepishly.

"Well, in the first place, that statement is perfectly consistent with innocence. That's just another way of saying, 'What have you got on me?' Maybe you don't know it, but his sister told him, right after the arrest, that unless the police found a weapon, they didn't have much of a case against him, or against anyone. Furthermore, you know as well as I do that statements made to a psychiatrist during a court-ordered examination cannot be introduced as evidence at the criminal trial. That would be self-incrimination."

"Yes, I suppose you're right."

"Then what is all this talk about other evidence?" Before he could respond, the clerk called the court to session.

Special Term Part I is, more often than not, a zoo. Any other word would be too charitable. Judges yell at lawyers, lawyers yell at judges, and the clerk yells at everybody. Occasionally a judge will insist on order and decorum, but usually chaos reigns. As one lawyer starts to say something, the other interrupts: "That's a lie. I never promised him that." The judge intercedes: "Let's hear from one of you at a time." And so it goes. With only minutes, sometimes seconds, available for each case, the lawyer's job is to say something, exaggerated or not, that will catch the judge's attention, make him forget there are 180 cases to be heard before lunch. If you do a good job, you might get as much as five or six minutes, sometimes more. In Special Term Part I, I always tell the judge I am a staff attorney at the Civil Liberties Union. Many judges do not like the Union, but at least they know it is not going to be another run-of-the-mill case.

So I trotted out my credentials and began, "The plaintiff in this case is an innocent man. The court of claims has already said so. But he is going to spend the rest of his life in Matteawan because the district attorney won't give him a chance to prove his innocence."

Judge Markowitz perked up a bit.

"The plaintiff has been found incompetent to stand trial on a felony charge. He wants to make a motion to dismiss the indictment, but under Code of Criminal Procedure section 662-b(3) he can't make *any* motions unless the D.A. consents, and he won't consent. We think that statute is unconstitutional."

Markowitz interrupted. "What's this about the court of claims?"

Good, he was interested. I told him briefly about the Orman decision. Then he leaned forward and said, "You know, I was a member of a bar committee that studied this problem, and, as I remember, we thought the statute should be changed." He paused and looked at us inquiringly. I said nothing; the assistant D.A. looked concerned. "Of course," the judge went on, "it's one thing to say a statute should be changed, and another to say that the Constitution requires it to be changed. What have you got to say about this?" He turned to the assistant D.A., who said what the state always says when it has a bad case on the merits— that the plaintiff "lacked standing to sue," and there was "no justiciable controversy." He closed on a stronger note: "Finally, I wish to point out that in the *Dickens* case, the appellate division [a higher court] held that this statute *is* constitutional. The court there said: 'Plainly, under section 662-b, dismissal of the indictment over the objection of the district attorney is not authorized. . . . Nor does petitioner indicate by what authority this court can compel the district attorney to withdraw his objection.' "

I was prepared for that; I had previously contacted the losing lawyer in that case and had spent several hours going over his file. "Your Honor," I said, "the *Dickens* case is clearly distinguishable. Although it is not evident from the opinion itself, it is clear from the record in that case that the incompetent defendant had asked the D.A. to consent to dismissal of the indictment—no more, no less. The court held, and properly so, that it could not order the D.A. to consent to dismissal of the indictment—that would be judicial interference with prosecutorial discretion. But we're not asking the D.A. to consent to dismissal. We're only asking that he consent to the *making of a motion* to dismiss. He could then oppose the granting of that motion on any grounds he wished. What we're asking does not in any sense interfere with prosecutorial discretion."

I could not tell if Markowitz thought the distinction was meaningful. Fearing reversal, most lower-court judges will not do anything a higher court has refused to do unless they see a strong basis for distinction.

That was it—time was up. We submitted our briefs and left the courtroom.

On March 19, I sent Teddy Neely a letter. He had sent me three—the latest wishing me a happy new year and "some sort of break on our case"—and I wanted to keep him informed.

Dear Mr. Neely:

This is just a note to let you know that we are still awaiting a decision from Judge Markowitz in your case. Evidently, he is giving it a great deal of thought. It's our feeling that the more time he spends thinking about your case, the greater the possibility that he'll see it our way. In any case, I will notify you the moment the decision comes down.

Three weeks later, I wrote another letter, this time to the judge.

Re: *Neely* v. *Hogan, et al.*
Index No. 18383/69

Dear Justice Markowitz:

It is my sad duty to inform you that the plaintiff in the above captioned class action died last Friday at Matteawan State Hospital. His relatives have asked me to do everything possible to facilitate adjudication of the issues raised in the complaint, as a tribute to his memory.

At 2:30 P.M. the preceding Friday, the elder Neely had called to tell me his son was dead. The telegram from Matteawan placed the time of death at 8:20 that morning. I could tell from his voice that Mr. Neely was deeply moved. Teddy, so long a patient, had been not a burden, not an embarrassment or annoyance, but a son whom he loved dearly. There was strength in his voice but also confusion. What had happened? How had he died? Only today his sister had received a cheerful letter from him. What had gone wrong? I told him I would call the superintendent of Matteawan, Dr. W. Cecil Johnston, and find out.

Dr. Johnston and I had, and continue to have, a strange relationship. We are not friends, though I have eaten at his table. Nor are we enemies, though I have opposed him, as director of Matteawan, more times than I can easily count. Although I disagree with virtually everything he says, I believe he is an honest man.

In my year and a half with the Civil Liberties Union, I had heard or seen ample evidence of cruel, even fatal, mistreatment in mental hospitals. I knew that mental patients were often beaten senseless by drunk or vicious attendants. Several hospital psychiatrists had come to my office to tell me so. (Within a month of Neely's death, two Matteawan guards were arrested and indicted for beating and kicking another Matteawan patient until he died.) I knew of a patient who had choked to death on her dinner because no hospital employees were around to pat her on the back. The hospital listed that one as a heart attack, but relatives had her hastily buried body dug up and an autopsy performed, and found the truth to be otherwise. I knew of one obstreperous patient who was first strapped to her bed by five attendants and who then had a wet pillowcase put over her head until she ceased to struggle. True, the attendants did not mean to kill her. The hospital director told the county medical examiner, "We would be satisfied with a report of 'death by exhaustion.'" I knew all these things, and more. I also knew that if Dr. Johnston told me there was nothing suspicious about Neely's death, I would believe him.

In minutes he was on the phone. Neely had come to the infirmary Thursday afternoon complaining of discomfort in his stomach. X rays showed nothing. When Neely fell into shock, Johnston went personally to the infirmary and began administering intravenous solutions, which Neely received throughout the night. Morning came, and with it Neely's death. Johnston told me he thought the cause of death was myocardial infarction—a heart attack—though he volunteered that the symptoms were not those a doctor would normally expect to find. Johnston had checked with the doctors, the guards, the other patients—there was no evidence that Neely had been injured or abused by anyone. Johnston was quite candid; he didn't know why Neely had died, but he was certain the cause of death was natural.

That was Friday. The funeral was set for Tuesday evening. Gwendolyn Lynch had asked me if I would come and "say a few words about Teddy." I was honored by her request, but also surprised. I had met Theodore Neely only three times; I hardly knew him. But on reflection I realized her request was not so surprising after all. For twenty years, patients had been Neely's only friends, and they could not attend his funeral. Except for his immediate family, I might be the only civilian with whom he had had any contact.

The M. Marshall Blake Funeral Home, at 10 St. Nicholas Place, near 150th Street, in Harlem, is a large old home with burnished wooden stairwells and creaking wooden floors. Off the small entrance hall to the left stands a comfortable old fireplace. To the right is a larger, longer room lined with folding chairs. At the end of that room was the coffin, covered tastefully with flowers. I found a seat near the back—the front was already full.

Most of the congregation were middle-aged or older—lifelong friends of Neely's parents, no doubt. Almost all were black. Gwendolyn Lynch came over to me, introduced her husband, and reminded me to say something about the lawsuit. All their friends had followed the news when Neely was arrested, she said, and most of them had assumed, reluctantly, that he was guilty. Very few knew anything about the Orman case or the proceedings still pending before Judge Markowitz. Gwendolyn Lynch took her place in the front row, between her mother and father, and the service began.

The minister seemed a kindly man, and it did not sound affected when he referred to the deceased as Teddy. He spoke in general terms, but I understood what he was saying. He was telling us that Neely's life had been more tragic by far than his death: the smartest kid in school, the target always for envy and abuse, looking forward to straight A's and a life loading trucks. No wonder he had found commune with the mad. And then, in 1952, lobotomy.

When it was my turn to speak, I briefly told a surprised congregation that Neely was an innocent man, that I had found him to be patient, but not resigned, and full of hope and dignity.

The next morning I wrote Judge Markowitz about Neely's death. Before the letter reached him, his law secretary called to tell me we had won. The opinion had been signed April 1, two days before Neely's death. In a scholarly ten-page opinion, Judge Markowitz adopted our distinction of the *Dickens* case, and held that an incompetent defendant "may make such motions addressed to the indictment as he may be advised without the consent of the District Attorney." The opinion ruled, sensibly, that incompetence suspends proceedings *against* a defendant, but not *by* him. Because of that decision, incompetent defendants are now able, through their attorneys, to make the kinds of motions competent defendants are able to make—motions to suppress illegally seized evidence, motions to preclude the use of illegally coerced confessions, motions to inspect grand jury minutes, motions to dismiss their indictments, and so on. The decision opened the courthouse door to incompetent defendants, for the first time giving them the opportunity for their day in court—an opportunity that brought hope to the hundreds still in Matteawan. One of them, a friend of Neely's, was Alfred Curt von Wolfersdorf. Neely's victory would mean a lot to him.

3 / Twenty Years in Matteawan

Cases like this could encourage the canard that Mr. Bumble was too generous by half when he suggested that "the law is a ass."

—THE HONORABLE MARVIN E. FRANKEL
United States District Judge

In early 1969, I received a letter from Alfred Curt von Wolfersdorf, an eighty-five-year-old patient at Matteawan State Hospital for the criminally insane. He had been at Matteawan almost twenty years.

In 1950, four unsolved murders had been committed in and around Poughkeepsie, New York, including the apparently senseless slaying of Bobby Leonard, a thirteen-year-old boy. According to von Wolfersdorf, "The police had to make an arrest to calm down the public and I, the landlord of the boy's family, was selected as a fall guy!" No one suggested that von Wolfersdorf was involved in the other three murders, and he pleaded not guilty to the Leonard charge. He never stood trial. Instead, he was found incompetent and committed to Matteawan "until he shall become sane, when he shall be returned to this court for disposition of the indictment pending against him."

There were about a thousand "incompetent" defendants at Matteawan, and 20 per cent of them had been confined, awaiting trial, even longer than von Wolfersdorf. The trial delay was of itself shocking, but the intriguing part of von Wolfersdorf's letter was his assertion that "two months after my arrest, the guilty man was found, tried, sentenced, and electrocuted in February, 1952, for killing the thirteen-year-old boy."

After months of investigation, including several trips to Poughkeepsie to examine old court records and newspaper archives, Loren Siegel and Lewis Novod, my two assistants, came up with documentary support for every one of von Wolfersdorf's allegations. His memory for events and conversations, some of them stretching over two decades, was perfect. Soon we were able to reconstruct the events following that October day in 1950 when two hunters found Bobby Leonard's body under a rotting mattress in an abandoned barn, a bullet through his head.

There was no apparent motive; Bobby had no money, no enemies. But he was dead, and no one knew who had shot him. Six weeks passed and still the police had no clues. Then, on December 1, 1950, Joe Paonessa telephoned the Dutchess County district attorney's office to implicate von Wolfersdorf. Paonessa pointed out that von Wolfersdorf was the landlord of the large frame house on High Street where Paonessa, Bobby, and Bobby's mother lived, and that years ago he had been a tenant on the DiRocco farm in Wappingers Falls where the dead boy's body was discovered. Why Paonessa made that call, no one will ever know. It would cost von Wolfersdorf his freedom, and Paonessa his life.

At midnight the following day, two detectives, acting on Paonessa's tip, roused the sixty-six-year-old von Wolfersdorf from bed and told him that Captain Brophy wanted to see him "right away" at the state troopers barracks. When he entered the barracks, says von Wolfersdorf, Captain Brophy called him a "lowdown, rotten, stinking son-of-a-bitch of a German bastard," and threatened to kill him if he did not confess. He was intermittently beaten and questioned by Captain Brophy and three officers until dawn. But von Wolfersdorf did not confess. Instead, he demanded a lie-detector test to establish his innocence. When the results of the test came back from Albany, the district attorney refused to disclose them and continued to hold von Wolfersdorf without bail.

Von Wolfersdorf's acquaintance with Bobby and his familiarity with the DiRocco farm were not of themselves sufficient to justify prosecution. The state's case against von Wolfersdorf depended upon the credibility of the only witness, Joe Paonessa.

It was strange that Paonessa should implicate von Wolfersdorf, perhaps his only friend. Von Wolfersdorf had felt sorry for Paonessa because he "never had a real house. His stepmother did not want him in the house because he was very untidy and a heavy drinker." At the request of Paonessa's father, an old friend and neighbor, von Wolfersdorf had permitted Paonessa to move into his own house, rent-free. Von Wolfersdorf bought Paonessa "a whole outfit of clothing, got him a job on the railroad in Coldspring, and he paid us back $5.00 a week for the clothes." But "as soon as Joe Paonessa had one drink, his will power was gone," and he lost job after job. Eventually, Paonessa began working on his own, repairing automobiles in the yard behind von Wolfersdorf's house. Bobby Leonard, who lived on the ground floor, "tried to make some spending money by helping Paonessa on repairing cars," but, said von Wolfersdorf, there were "quite a lot of arguments between those two" because "the boy was not satisfied with a dollar a week, while Paonessa pocketed $36 and $40 in one business."

On January 30, 1951, two months after his telephone tip, Paonessa accompanied the authorities to the scene of the crime and told them that while he sat in an automobile some distance away, von Wolfersdorf had murdered Bobby Leonard. But after questioning by District Attorney W. Vincent Grady, Paonessa broke down and admitted he had shot the boy himself. He claimed, however, that von Wolfersdorf had given him a gun (a claim he later recanted) and a sealed note signed "Red" telling him to "take care of Bobby." The handwriting, he was certain, was not von Wolfersdorf's.

There were many strange things about Joe Paonessa. Not the least of them was the frequency with which he changed his story and his aplomb in shrugging off allegations of inconsistency. In some versions, Paonessa was present at the crime; in others, he was waiting in the car, or in an adjacent shack, or in a tavern thirty-five miles away. But the police listened to him, even when he claimed that von Wolfersdorf, though not present at the crime, had ruled his actions by "thought control."

On February 5, 1951, the grand jury indicted both Paonessa and von Wolfersdorf for murder and kidnapping. Six weeks later, the district attorney requested a sanity examination for von Wolfersdorf, though not, inexplicably, for Paonessa. Whatever the D.A.'s motivation, von Wolfersdorf was committed to Harlem Valley State Hospital, in Wingdale, New York, to be examined by Doctors Ernest S. Steblen and Charles A. Angelo.

Their eighteen-page report indicates the notoriety of the case (most defendants get a page or two at most), and illustrates the inability of psychiatrists to think in legal terms. If a lawyer were asked to prepare a psychiatric evaluation of a defendant, he would refuse, admitting that he knew little about psychiatry. Psychiatrists, on the other hand, know little about the law, yet when asked to evaluate a defendant's competence to stand trial, a legal question, they invariably comply—or think they do. Nowhere in the report of Doctors Steblen and Angelo is there a word about von Wolfersdorf's ability to assist counsel in preparing a defense or his ability to understand the nature of the charges against him, the two indispensable requirements of a competent defendant.

What is required of a defendant varies enormously from case to case. In some, the defendant must testify; in others, his lawyer may be able to establish a defense without subjecting the defendant to the risks of cross-examination. Some trials involve complex factual issues that the defendant will have to help his attorney untangle; in others, the facts are undisputed or available from disinterested third parties. Frequently, the only issues are legal issues, requiring little or no help from the defendant. Only the defense attorney knows with any certainty how much information and assistance from the defendant the case will require. Psychiatrists do not know, for example, whether the trial will require the defendant's co-operation for thirty days or for thirty minutes. A defendant may be quite capable of making a reasoned decision to plead guilty, but not sufficiently stable to withstand a complex and prolonged trial. But only the defendant and his attorney know whether he will stand trial or plead guilty. In short, psychiatrists are less able to make a meaningful evaluation of a defendant's competence to stand trial (or plead guilty) than are defense attorneys.

Perhaps that is why psychiatrists so often resolve the legal issues by ignoring them. Instead of trying to think in legal terms, they stick to their own field, deciding whether or not the defendant is mentally ill or psychotic, and assuming—incorrectly—that if he is either, he must be incompetent to stand trial, as Dr. Abrahamsen had in the Youngblood case. Thus Doctors Steblen and Angelo reasoned that "because of this man's psychosis we believe that he is, at the time of this examination, in such a state of insanity as to be incapable of understanding the charge against him, or the proceedings, or of making his defense"—even though they had asked him no questions about the charge, the proceedings, or possible defenses.

The two psychiatrists found von Wolfersdorf to be "a man of superior intelligence," with a good memory. He was "co-operative, pleasant, and sociable," "very neat and clean," gave "good attention," and neither heard voices nor saw visions. In fact, the doctors were hard-pressed to find anything wrong with von Wolfersdorf. The main rationale for their finding of psychosis, which they stressed again and again, was his "absurd thoughts regarding a secret society" known as the Civil and Political Correction Service.

The psychiatrists reported von Wolfersdorf's assertion that his first contact with the society was in late 1928, when "we had a heavy snow and we could not get out for four days." Then "some people came and plowed our alley," and a laconic man "who called himself 'Red' " gave von Wolfersdorf "a big box of groceries." "Red" explained that the society was still "undercover," and that its purpose was "to help poor people" and to overthrow "the crooked politicians." Months, and sometimes years, would pass between chance encounters with "Red," who occasionally asked von Wolfersdorf to deliver sealed envelopes to other persons, including Paonessa.

Von Wolfersdorf's belief in a secret society is strange, even bizarre, but that does not mean it is necessarily incorrect and therefore evidence of psychosis. Paonessa, too, believed in the Civil and Political Correction Service and in "Red"; and his lawyer, Stephen Bienick, explained to reporters that the society was "an extension of the German-American Bund." No one called them crazy. Even before Doctors Steblen and Angelo prepared their report, District Attorney Grady had confirmed the existence of "Red" and identified him as Clifford "Red" Zimmerman, a former Poughkeepsie house painter. Grady took statements from Zimmerman, then in Sing Sing prison serving a sentence for forgery, in which Zimmerman admitted he had known von Wolfersdorf for several years. Nevertheless, because of his "absurd beliefs," von Wolfersdorf was found incompetent. On May 25,

1951, John R. Schwartz, Dutchess County judge, committed him to Matteawan.*

In May of 1970, almost twenty years after von Wolfersdorf had been hospitalized because of his "absurd beliefs," Loren, Lewis and I made the sixty-mile trip to Matteawan for our first meeting with him. As he was led into a five-by-seven-foot interview cubicle by an armed guard (who planted himself just outside the open door), I noted his impeccable dress—navy blue shirt, gray pin-striped suit (the wide lapels were now in style again), tastefully flowered tie, gray sideburns, and trim mustache. His manner was polite, austere, and very European. He spoke quietly with a heavy German accent. He was eighty-six years old, but he looked no more than seventy. He had not confessed to any involvement in the crime even though, according to his wife, "he was advised to 'forget all' until he admitted" guilt. And the stigma of "mental illness" seemed hardly to have touched him, so staunchly did he believe in his own sanity.

Von Wolfersdorf told us that he rarely had any contact with psychiatrists and was interviewed only when scheduled for another of his court appearances (he periodically asked the courts to find him competent, so he could stand trial), an allegation that was supported by his hospital record. On August 18, 1952, a doctor had entered a one-paragraph note about von Wolfersdorf in the hospital record. The next entry, also one paragraph, was

---

* People are frequently labeled mad because psychiatrists discredit true, but seemingly bizarre, stories. In one reported case, a man spent four years at Matteawan because the psychiatrists thought he suffered from a delusion: he claimed to have seen his wife's lover slash his wrists, drain the blood into a beer mug, and drink it. The psychiatrists did not bother to investigate that claim, but a lawyer finally did. The wife confirmed under oath that her husband's "delusion" was, in fact, true, and four days later he was discharged from Matteawan. A similar case of a psychiatric diagnosis based in large part on the psychiatrist's disbelief in the underlying facts is described in the next chapter.

dated October 22, 1953, fourteen months later—and so the pattern was set. Under the date of August 10, 1960, I found the following "interview" report:

When he came for interview he said he has nothing to change or add to what he said previously. On the ward he is reported as being clean and neat, quiet, agreeable, sociable with others, interested in ward activities, works in the patients' clothes room, and is a good worker.

The next entry, dated December 9, 1961, sixteen months later, was a three-sentence note reporting that von Wolfersdorf had been transferred to a different ward for "closer supervision." He had somehow managed to smuggle out a letter "without passing through the regular channels." The next entry, another one-paragraph report of an "interview," was dated March 16, 1962, or nineteen months after the previous one. He was scheduled for a court hearing on March 22; hence the need for the March 16 interview. After all, the doctors could not very well appear in court on March 22 and swear to von Wolfersdorf's continued incompetence if they had not even talked to him for nineteen months. The March 22 hearing was adjourned, which required another interview on April 26, 1962. On September 10, 1963, seventeen months later, a doctor reported "no improvement since last examination on April 26, 1962." What had prompted the September 10 interview? Was it because on September 13 von Wolfersdorf was scheduled for yet another judicial hearing?

Our meeting confirmed what his letters had suggested: von Wolfersdorf was quite competent to stand trial. There was no doubt about it. But I knew that on sixteen separate occasions he had requested a judicial determination of competence and had lost every time, usually without a hearing. Future competency hearings would be before the same judges who had turned him down so many times in the past. No hope there. Then an idea began to form—what did it matter whether he was competent or not? Even if he was competent, he could not be brought to trial.

The only "evidence" the state had had to link von Wolfersdorf to the crime was the testimony of Joe Paonessa. And two years after the murder, Paonessa had been convicted and electrocuted.

Even before Paonessa's death, the state's case against von Wolfersdorf had been weak—the self-contradictory story of a co-defendant who had a clear motive to implicate von Wolfersdorf and thereby reduce his own guilt. After Paonessa's death, the state had no case at all. For eighteen years von Wolfersdorf had been confined to Matteawan because he was incompetent to stand trial, even though, had he been competent, the state could not possibly have proved his guilt. I could argue that von Wolfersdorf's confinement, based as it was on the fiction that he would someday be brought to trial, violated his constitutional right to "due process of law" and to a "speedy trial." And I could argue that confinement at Matteawan, a prisonlike hospital for the *criminally* insane, was so incompatible with the presumption of innocence as to constitute a "cruel and unusual punishment."

I wanted to make those arguments before a federal judge—we wouldn't stand a chance in state court. But before filing a federal habeas corpus petition it is necessary to exhaust state court remedies. (Theoretically, state courts can vindicate constitutional rights; with few exceptions, they rarely do.) The ordinary procedure, for a competent defendant, would be to move to dismiss the indictment in a state court. But, as has been noted, under state law incompetent defendants were not then permitted to challenge their indictments unless the D.A. consented, which he customarily refused to do. Von Wolfersdorf was in the same situation as Theodore Neely, whose case I was working on at the time. Neely's case was stronger, so I suspended work on von Wolfersdorf and pushed ahead on Neely. Within a few months, I was able to file a motion to dismiss von Wolfersdorf's indictment, relying on the Neely decision as authority to make the motion whether the D.A. consented or not.

Upon arrival in Poughkeepsie, I discovered that the supreme

court judge who was to decide the motion was the same W. Vincent Grady who, as district attorney, had obtained the indictment against von Wolfersdorf twenty years earlier. Remarking that von Wolfersdorf was "quite a character," Judge Grady disqualified himself and transferred the motion to the county court.

The county court judges were too busy that day to hear oral argument. I could either submit the motion for decision on the basis of the written materials before the court or I could wait another month and present oral argument. Since I knew we could not win in state court, and, in any event, my only purpose was to go through the routine of exhausting state court remedies and get into federal court, I decided to submit.

I drove back from Poughkeepsie and began to draft the pleadings and brief for a federal habeas corpus proceeding. On July 25, 1970, I learned that the county court had, as expected, denied the motion. And just in time. Habeas corpus proceedings were heard in the federal court in New York City on Tuesday afternoons. Judge Marvin E. Frankel would be sitting on the afternoon of Tuesday, August 11, 1970, for one day only. Two years earlier, he had written a decision in which he found a twelve-year delay in the trial of a competent defendant to be "patently shocking on its face." With Judge Frankel, we might have a chance. I filed the papers and waited.

At 9:00 A.M. on the eleventh, I checked the *New York Law Journal* and found, to my dismay, that von Wolfersdorf was not listed among the cases to be argued at 2:15 that afternoon. The clerk assured me over the telephone that the case would no doubt be on the official calendar posted outside the courtroom. At two o'clock I arrived and scanned the official calendar. Not there. I dashed down the hall to the clerk's office and pestered an assistant clerk until, obviously annoyed, he walked back with me to the courtroom and added "*United States ex rel. Alfred Curt von Wolfersdorf* v. *W. C. Johnston*," in ink, to the bottom of the typed calendar.

At 2:15, the clerk began calling the calendar to see if the lawyers were ready to argue. When he came to von Wolfersdorf, an assistant attorney general announced that he was going to ask Judge Frankel for a one- or two-week adjournment so that he could study the case. I introduced myself to the assistant and asked to speak to him in the hall. He was young, and seemed nervous and inexperienced, so I tried to sound affronted as I reminded him of the court rule that requests for adjournments should be made by noon of the day preceding argument—knowing, as I gambled he did not, that the rule was more often ignored than followed. I then suggested that if he would agree to proceed that day with a short oral argument, I would allow him until Monday, the seventeenth, to submit opposing papers. He wasn't persuaded. "That wouldn't be too bad, but I'm still going to ask for an adjournment," he said, and we returned to the courtroom.

I knew that if he asked for an adjournment, he would get it, and I would lose Judge Frankel. Normally, the attorney applying for an adjournment speaks first, but, relying on his inexperience, I took the initiative and stepped to the lectern.

Your Honor, my name is Bruce J. Ennis. I am a staff attorney with the New York Civil Liberties Union, and as such I represent the relator in this habeas corpus proceeding brought to challenge the constitutionality of his twenty-year confinement at Matteawan State Hospital. I have been informed that the state would prefer an adjournment. However, I just spoke with the assistant attorney general and I believe it may be acceptable to argue the matter today with leave to the state to file papers on or before this coming Friday.

"No," interjected the assistant. "You said Monday."

He was trapped. I could not have hoped to provoke a more exploitable response. Before he could continue, I resumed, "Monday will be perfectly acceptable to the relator."

So much for the adjournment; now on to the merits. I began my argument as I had begun my brief:

The question raised by this petition can be simply stated. Let us suppose a man is charged with crime. Let us suppose he is innocent. Let us suppose, also, that he is incompetent to prove his innocence. Can he constitutionally be held, under criminal auspices, for twenty years? That is what the state has done to this relator. That is what we ask this court to change.

I could tell Judge Frankel was interested. I could also tell that he was troubled by something. Finally he interrupted me. "I do not seem to have the papers in this case."

The petition had been added to the calendar so hastily that the judge's copies of the papers were still in the clerk's office. In order to forestall a renewed suggestion of adjournment, I immediately offered to hand the judge my personal copies, and he accepted. Because of his unfamiliarity with the case, I was able to argue at somewhat greater length than is normally permitted. After discussion of the facts and law, I concluded:

Perhaps it would be unfair to bring relator to trial. But is it fair to confine him until he dies in a hospital for the "criminally" insane, simply because he is incompetent to prove his innocence? If it is, then we must admit to ourselves that the presumption of innocence means nothing; that an allegation of crime, no matter how spurious, is equivalent to proof of crime. That cannot be the law.

The assistant rose in opposition. He had not uttered three words before he was interrupted by a question from the bench:

Q. Is it true that this man is eighty-six years old?
A. Yes, Your Honor.
Q. Is it true that he has been hospitalized for almost twenty years?

A. Yes, Your Honor.

Q. Well, let me say that I am overwhelmingly disposed to grant this petition, but let me hear what you have to say.

That was it! We were going to win! I sat back to listen.

After a few minutes, the judge interrupted the assistant again. "I am going to tell you something because I am a lot older than you." He described the state's objections to our petition as "technical." So far, so good. Then came the bombshell:

Q. Have you discussed this case with Mr. Lefkowitz [the attorney general of the state of New York]?

A. No, Your Honor, I have not.

Q. Well, I suggest you get in touch with him and see if he really wants to oppose this petition, because if he does, I will have to write an opinion.

The handwriting was on the wall. The judge had as much as told the state that if it did not voluntarily release von Wolfersdorf from Matteawan, he would be released by court order. My eighteen months of work on the case would come to nothing. The state would back down and agree to release von Wolfersdorf, but what of the thousands of defendants like him all over the country? There would be no decision, no precedent to help them. I was disappointed, though not surprised. Civil liberties and civil rights lawyers learn quickly that many state and federal judges will do everything they can to avoid publicly criticizing "the authorities." As a consequence, government agencies can and frequently do adopt positions that are legally untenable, or even frivolous, knowing full well that if the issue is ever forced to a decision, the judge will almost certainly warn the agency it is going to lose and allow it to withdraw graciously, without judicial criticism.

Recently, for example, in a case handled by my office, a federal appellate judge was so outraged by the government's groundless defense of a civil liberties case that he turned to the assistant United States attorney and said, "Is there no one in the executive department with the courage to do justice?" Then, instead of issuing an order, the court gave the government twenty-four hours to change its mind, which it did. The case was then dismissed as moot. Nine months later, because it was under no judicial mandate to the contrary, the government reverted to its original position, forcing the plaintiff to start again at the bottom of the judicial ladder. The reverse never happens. Never does the judge turn to the ACLU or the NAACP and say, "I think your case is frivolous. I advise you to withdraw your complaint or I will write a decision that you may not like to have on the books." He simply writes the decision.

There was nothing I could do but wait for the inevitable. The judge had given the attorney general six days either to change his mind about bringing von Wolfersdorf to trial or to specify, under oath, "the nature of the evidence upon which the People would propose to proceed in such a trial." Inexplicably, the attorney general did neither. Instead, he "requested that relator's application in all respects be denied," even while conceding "it is possible that the indictment against the relator might be dismissed if he was in fact able to stand trial."

I still do not know why the attorney general refused to capitulate. Perhaps, as I was informally told, it had something to do with the "bad feeling" in the community about von Wolfersdorf (years before, 250 residents of Dutchess County had petitioned Governor Thomas E. Dewey to spare Paonessa's life, alleging that Paonessa was only a "tool" under the "domination" of von Wolfersdorf). Perhaps, because 1970 was an election year, the attorney general did not want to be held responsible for releasing the alleged murderer of a thirteen-year-old boy. Whatever the reason, the state's ambiguous response did not satisfy Judge Frankel, and he ordered a more specific reply. Within hours, the assistant attorney general submitted a supplemental affidavit:

> Upon information supplied by the Dutchess County District Attorney, [my] statement in Court that there was evidence upon which the relator could be tried was incorrect. Due to the loss of key witnesses such as the codefendant and the passage of time it would, according to the District Attorney's office, be highly unlikely that the petitioner could be brought to trial if he was found able to stand trial in the near future.

The state had finally admitted that it had what Judge Frankel characterized as "no speck of evidence" against von Wolfersdorf. Yet even now, with no evidence, the state still refused to drop the criminal charges against von Wolfersdorf, and even refused to transfer him to a civil hospital. Within the month, Judge Frankel ordered the state to release von Wolfersdorf from Matteawan.

What must it be like to be governed for twenty years by men who believe you have committed the most serious of crimes, and believe you mad because you claim to be innocent? A similar question must have prompted Judge Frankel to preface his decision with a description of Matteawan as "a place more likely to drive men mad than to cure the 'insane.' " The decision itself was a masterpiece; we could not have asked for more. After brushing aside the state's procedural objections by citing the *Neely* case, Judge Frankel turned to the merits, adopting each of the three constitutional arguments we had urged, though in reverse order:

(1) Relator's incarceration among the "criminally insane" for 20 years because of his status as an insane defendant (presumed innocent) named in an untriable indictment violates his protection against cruel and unusual punishment as it is enforceable against the States under the Fourteenth Amendment. . . .

(2) Without the specific ban of the Eighth Amendment [cruel and unusual punishment], the shocking circumstances of relator's

imprisonment would violate the Due Process Clause of the Fourteenth Amendment · · .

(3) Relator's counsel argues that the pending state indictment must be deemed a nullity because a trial upon it now would violate his [Sixth Amendment] right to a speedy trial. . . . Notwithstanding that the delay has not been the State's "fault," the argument is powerful. . . . The court adopts it, but solely as additional ground for the specific decision herein. That is to say . . . this court does not purport in more general terms to "dismiss" or otherwise erase the indictment. If the State should ever undertake to bring relator to trial, today's decision is not meant to foreclose (however much it may predict defeat of) a prosecution claim that such proceedings are consistent with the right to a speedy trial. All this court now holds, or needs to hold, is that for purposes of the concrete claim to elementary decency now ripe for decision, the implications of the federal right to have an indictment tried and done with forbid the gruesome use to which the State has put its pending charge.

Thus, in one stroke, a federal court had ruled, for the first time anywhere in the United States, that incompetent state court defendants are entitled to the protections of the Sixth, Eighth, and Fourteenth Amendments to the Constitution. The ruling was important in itself, but even more important for what it presaged.

The first ground of decision, for example, considerably expands the utility of the Eighth Amendment as a preconviction remedy even for "sane" defendants. Since the purpose of preconviction confinement is not to punish the defendant, but only to ensure his presence at trial, the state should not be permitted to curtail the rights of a preconviction defendant any more than is necessary to make sure he will appear on the trial date. Therefore, preconviction restrictions (mail censorship and the like) and conditions of confinement must be less onerous than postconviction restrictions and conditions or they will be subject to attack as

"punishment" for the mere status of being charged with crime—
a punishment incompatible with the presumption of innocence.
For "insane" defendants, the ruling probably means they will
have to be hospitalized, if at all, in civil hospitals, not with the
criminally insane.

The second ground suggests that incompetent but presumably
innocent defendants may have the right to stand trial as incompetents before they can be hospitalized involuntarily. If the state
cannot make out a criminal case against them, there is nothing
they need be competent for; if it can, then and only then can the
defendant be hospitalized, with the right upon restoration of
competence to assert any alibi or other defense that, because of
his incompetence, he was unable to assert at his previous trial.

The third ground may prove to be the most important. Substantial trial delay is always prejudicial to a defendant. Witnesses
die, memories fade, and documents are lost, whether the defendant is competent or not. The right to a speedy trial is an ancient
and fundamental right, and one that is no less important when
the defendant is insane. For more than eight hundred years, the
principle that justice delayed is justice denied has been a corner-
stone of Anglo-American jurisprudence. Judge Frankel recognized that the guarantee of a speedy trial protects rights of such
fundamental importance that it must be honored even when the
state's purpose in delaying trial is ostensibly humane. How much
more is that ruling required when the incompetency proceeding
is begun for less honorable motives. The last paragraph of our
reply memorandum put it this way:

All too often prosecutors invoke incompetency proceedings, over
the defendant's objection, as a dispositional alternative to criminal
trial. If successful, the prosecution obtains the results of a criminal
conviction (incarceration) without giving the defendant the procedural protections of a criminal trial (jury trial, proof beyond a reasonable doubt, etc.). Sometimes the prosecutor is motivated by

humane considerations. Frequently, however, incompetency proceedings are invoked simply because the prosecution does not have enough evidence to convict. Prosecutors are much less likely to abuse their discretion to invoke incompetency proceedings if they know that after a finite period of time, the Sixth Amendment right to a speedy trial will require dismissal of the criminal charges. That is what we ask this Court to hold.

And that, in principle, is what the court did hold.

Within a week of the decision, von Wolfersdorf was transferred to a civil mental hospital in Binghamton, New York. I waited a month, to be sure the state would not appeal, and then telephoned the hospital and asked to speak with his supervising psychiatrist, who told me that von Wolfersdorf was "alert, cooperative and happy," and was "not causing any problems." In fact, the hospital was "ready to discharge him as soon as suitable arrangements in the community" could be found. What a miraculous improvement! Twenty years at Matteawan and he was still considered too crazy to stand trial. One month in a civil hospital and he was ready for the community. There is an important point here: psychiatric evaluations are not scientific, are not even medical in any meaningful sense of that term. Insanity, like beauty, is in the eye of the beholder. This is not to say that there are no verbal or behavioral phenomena that can be observed, categorized, and related to statistical norms. It is to say that those phenomena may or may not be labeled insane, depending on the cultural background and the personal beliefs and values of the examiner. Von Wolfersdorf's astonishing recovery reflects the enormous philosophical gap between penal psychiatrists and civil psychiatrists—no more, no less.

The next step, of course, was to get von Wolfersdorf out of the civil hospital and back to the community. The hospital authorities were willing to discharge him, but they were not legally authorized to do so until the criminal charges against him had been dropped.

On April 20, 1971, I went back to the county court and renewed the motion to dismiss the indictment. This time I was able to point out that a federal judge had found there was no evidence against von Wolfersdorf, a fact that the attorney general had conceded. As I rose to present oral argument, I could tell that the county judge, Raymond E. Aldrich, Jr., could barely suppress his irritation—his face was literally flushed with emotion. Finally, unable to contain himself longer, he blurted, "What right does a federal court have to order the state to reveal its evidence in a criminal case?" I told Judge Aldrich that the federal court's power to do what it had done was no longer an issue. If the state had wanted to resist Judge Frankel's order to reveal the state's evidence, it could have appealed his order to a higher court, but it had not. The important point was that the attorney general *had* complied with that order and had admitted, under oath, that the state had no evidence against von Wolfersdorf.

Judge Aldrich then made a remarkable statement. He told me he was not going to pay any attention to the attorney general's affidavit because the district attorney, a county official, and not the attorney general, a state official, was in charge of the prosecution against von Wolfersdorf. When I asked what difference that made, Judge Aldrich replied heatedly that the district attorney might have some evidence the attorney general did not know about. I pointed out that the attorney general had expressly based his affidavit "upon information supplied by the Dutchess County District Attorney," but even that did not dissuade Judge Aldrich. It was impossible to reason with him, so I left the courtroom.

On June 28, 1971, two months later, I received Judge Aldrich's decision. As expected, it denied our motion to dismiss the indictment. I had hoped that if Aldrich would neither dismiss the indictment nor direct the D.A., in addition to the attorney general, to reveal all of the state's evidence, he would at least order the

D.A. to demonstrate that the state had *some* evidence. But he would not do even that: "This court will not require the people to come forward and reveal at this time evidence even to make out a prima facie case."

I could not appeal Judge Aldrich's decision, because under state law the denial of a motion to dismiss an indictment is not appealable. The theory is that the defendant will be promptly brought to trial on the charge, and if convicted he can appeal his conviction, raising the same issues as in his motion to dismiss the indictment. The theory breaks down, of course, when applied to incompetent defendants, because they will not be brought to trial at all. I wanted to challenge the nonappealability rule as applied to incompetents, but this was not the proper case for making that challenge. Appeals from the Dutchess County Court go to the Appellate Division, Third Department (New York is divided into four appellate court regions), and that court was particularly antagonistic to cases brought by mental patients.

Since any further state court proceedings on behalf of von Wolfersdorf would be futile, I began to consider other approaches. The obvious answer was to have von Wolfersdorf declared competent to stand trial. Then the state would have to try him, and it was inconceivable that a jury would convict. If he won the criminal trial, he would be free. If, by some chance, he lost, the worst that could happen would be a sentence of life imprisonment (subsequent to Paonessa's electrocution, New York had abolished the death penalty)—a sentence he was already in effect serving.

I called a few people I knew in the headquarters of the state Department of Mental Hygiene, and a few weeks later von Wolfersdorf was re-examined and found to be competent.

On September 13, 1971, Louis Dozoretz, the director of the hospital where von Wolfersdorf was then confined, wrote to Albert M. Rosenblatt, the district attorney for Dutchess County, explaining that von Wolfersdorf had recovered and was now competent to stand trial. I received a copy of that letter on October 7, and on the twelfth I wrote Rosenblatt to suggest we have a pretrial conference—I was still hopeful that, faced at last with the prospect of a trial, the D.A. would relent and drop the charges. He replied that he had never received the Dozoretz letter. Several weeks and four telephone calls from my office later, Dozoretz finally sent another letter to the D.A.

On November 30, 1971, I wrote a second time to the D.A., again requesting a pretrial conference. My letter was not answered, and the assistant D.A. in charge of the case refused for weeks to accept or return my repeated telephone calls. Finally, after I told his secretary one day that I *knew* he was there, the assistant D.A. picked up the phone and said that if I would make a third motion to dismiss the indictment, his office "might" consent to dismissal. I made the motion on January 20, 1972, returnable before Judge Aldrich on February 8. On February 3, the D.A. filed an affidavit consenting, "in the interest of justice," to dismissal.

Ordinarily, a D.A.'s consent will be sufficient to persuade a court to dismiss an indictment. But it was not enough for Judge Aldrich. Two months later, he denied our third motion to dismiss and ordered the D.A. to prosecute von Wolfersdorf. I called the D.A., who said he was "puzzled" by Judge Aldrich's decision, and then set to work again. Von Wolfersdorf's murder trial would be my first criminal case, and I had a lot to learn before then. For his part, eighty-eight-year-old Alfred Curt von Wolfersdorf did what he had done for more than twenty years; he accepted the bad news and waited.*

* Neely was dead and von Wolfersdorf was still waiting, but their cases would mean a lot to others. On June 7, 1972, in *Jackson* v. *Indiana*, the United States Supreme Court greatly expanded the rights of allegedly incompetent defendants, citing *Neely* and *von Wolfersdorf* as grounds for its decision.

4 / Paranoia

There was little to do in Green Haven Prison except write letters, but Jerome Wright wrote one too many. On December 4, 1968, the night before he was to be paroled, having served five years of a three-and-a-half-to-seven-year sentence for carrying a concealed, loaded pistol, Wright scribbled to his mother what Warden Harold Follette considered to be a "paranoic-type letter" in which Wright claimed his life was in danger.

We do not know exactly what the letter said, because Warden Follette was unable to produce it on request. We do know that if Wright had not written it, he would have been freed. Instead,

Follette canceled his parole and had him examined by two psychiatrists, who agreed that Wright was paranoid and transferred him to Dannemora State Hospital—250 miles north of Stormville, New York, where Green Haven is located.

Characterized by a federal judge as a "restrictive prison," Dannemora is a hospital operated by the Department of Corrections for convicted prisoners who have become mentally ill while in prison. Dannemora's isolated location near the Canadian border, thirty miles from the nearest public transportation, curtailed visits from Wright's friends and relatives, but it did not curb his penchant for letter writing.

Hello Mom,

How are you and Dad feeling today? I am feeling well and I sincerely hope that this letter finds you both feeling well and in the very best of health.

I presume you received a copy of the papers committing me to the State Hospital. I did not write you before now because I was waiting until I saw the doctors. However, I have been here five days and I have not spoken to a psychiatrist except very briefly the day that I came in. Therefore, I really don't have very much to tell you except that I am here at the Dannemora State Hospital in Plattsburgh, New York. My new number is 8209.

How is Ann, Charles, and the children doing? The next time that you see or speak to them plese tell them hello for me and that I wish them a happy holiday season. Tell Ann that I will write her as soon as I can get some stamps. My stamps from Green Haven should be here in a few days.

All I want you to send me is a package with some apples and nuts. (I asked the officer if we are allowed to have *nuts* in here) (smile).

With all my love,
Your son, Jerome Wright
#8209.

Jerome was right; his mother had received a copy of the papers committing him to Dannemora, and had asked me to get him out. It was my first day at the Civil Liberties Union, and I knew very little about mental patients and the law, probably no more than the average lawyer. But I had read enough to know that in *Baxstrom v. Herold*, a case involving another Dannemora inmate, the United States Supreme Court had ruled that upon expiration of his prison sentence Johnnie K. Baxstrom had to be released from Dannemora and transferred to the less restrictive facilities of a civil mental hospital. Although Wright's sentence had not expired, he had been scheduled for parole, and it seemed to me that the principle was the same: when there is no longer a penal justification for incarceration—whether because of expiration of sentence or because of recommendation for parole—then the individual should be treated as a civilian; if mentally ill, he should go to a civil mental hospital, not an institution like Dannemora.

Mrs. Wright requested judicial review of the transfer to Dannemora. On December 27, the Wrights and I made the two-hour trip to Poughkeepsie, where the hearing was to be held. Without telling us, however, the judge had decided to extend his holiday into the new year, so the hearing was rescheduled for January 17, 1969, at Green Haven.

After signing in at the security desk and walking forward and back and forward again through the metal-detecting arch, I was escorted to a small room where, for the first time, I met Jerome Wright, back from Dannemora for the trial. He was a shy, slight man of about thirty. As we talked I became increasingly uneasy. I had not planned to contest the factual allegation that Jerome Wright was mentally ill. I had planned to raise only a straightforward legal issue, contending that even if he was mentally ill, he had the right to be transferred from Dannemora to a civil hospital. But Jerome Wright did not seem at all crazy, and I saw no reason for him to be in any hospital, prison or civil. True, he was fearful, but his fears were not mere fantasies—other prisoners had *told* him that because he was considered to be an informer, his life was in danger.

"Mr. Wright, can you tell me the names of some of the prisoners who told you that?"

"No."

"Why not?"

"Well, if it ever got back that I used their names, then I would really be in trouble."

"Look, you've got to tell me their names so I can call them as witnesses, or we're going to lose. It's as simple as that. If it's just your word, we don't stand a chance."

He thought for a long time. "I'm sorry. I just can't tell you."

I had twenty minutes until the trial—twenty minutes to prepare a factual defense I had not even expected to raise. That was not enough time even to read through Wright's prison record, but I read what I could and then headed upstairs to the courtroom.

Thomas Dorsey, an assistant attorney general with several years' experience on the "mental hygiene" docket, called as his first witness Dr. Robert C. Humme, chief of the Male Admission Service at Hudson River State Hospital, a mental hospital ten miles east of Green Haven. Humme testified that on December 11, 1968, he had examined Jerome Wright and had concluded "that he suffers from paranoid schizophrenia, [and] that he would benefit by psychiatric hospitalization."

On cross-examination, I asked Dr. Humme to give specific examples of Wright's paranoia.

Be glad to. He is afraid of informants who have talked about him, and he states, "I was told by" an associate or friend "that I am suspected of being an informer." . . . He states it is possible that officers or hospital personnel could be bribed, "they could try to kill me," but in stating this he shows no emotional affect, no evidence of fear.

"Affect" is a psychiatric term used to describe a person's emotional response to the world around him. If he laughs when telling a sad story, or cries when he hears good news, his affect may be considered inappropriate, or out of tune with the real world. Many psychiatrists believe that inappropriate affect is a sign of mental illness. Dr. Humme initially testified that Wright's affect was "flat," and therefore "inappropriate," because he described threats to his life in a calm, matter-of-fact way. Later Dr. Humme admitted that he would still have characterized Wright's narrative as inappropriate even if he had related "the same information, but had done so in a more concerned and fearful manner." Why? Because, in Dr. Humme's words, "my knowledge of this prison is that it is well run and that his danger is minimal." In other words, it was not so much Wright's nonchalant manner of expressing concern for his safety that was inappropriate as the fact that he was concerned at all. That his concern was based not on hallucinations but on statements made by other prisoners was, in Dr. Humme's view, irrelevant.

Q. Let us assume that the statements made by the other prisoners are totally without basis, that they do not themselves have any real basis for saying that Jerome Wright's life is in danger, nevertheless, for whatever reason they made those statements to him, would that not be a reasonable basis and a rational basis for him to act upon them?

A. I can specifically state this would not change my opinion if other prisoners have told him that he is in danger.

A few minutes later, Dr. Humme insisted on volunteering another example of inappropriate affect.

A. When I asked him this morning what would he do if he was released, he said, "Outside I'd sit around and have a drink and laugh about it." This was said without emotion, without appropriate affect, and seems to me to be a totally inappropriate and psychotic reaction.

Q. And why is that?

A. Because for a patient, an individual who is so fearful while protected to say that when released, which he apparently seeks, that he would then sit around and take a drink and laugh about it, is inappropriate, illogical, and is evidence of mental illness in my professional opinion.

Q. Doctor, if the persons he is afraid of are themselves in a prison, and if he fears for his safety only because he is in a prison with those inmates, would it not be perfectly rational to feel secure and safe if he was removed from a prison where those inmates could hurt him?

A. I don't agree with that, no. I think a person who is as disturbed and fearful as this man could be fearful outside, and I would not have much credence in that statement "if I," in quotes, "if I were released, I would just sit around, take a drink, and laugh about it."

So far, the state's case seemed to me unpersuasive. Perhaps Dorsey agreed. On redirect examination he tried to bolster the diagnosis:

Q. Now, Doctor, in answer to some of Mr. Ennis's questions you discussed some of the fears that the patient displayed when you interviewed him. I ask you if there were any other irrational fears that he had?

A. Yes. He was offered a cigarette in a courtesy, and he said, "No, I don't smoke. I stopped two years ago." He said this without affect, inappropriate affect, and I asked, "Why was that?" and he said, "Because it says on the cigarette package smoking may be harmful to me." That means that he is confusing the danger of cigarette smoking, which is enjoyed by many people, even prisoners, with his unreal fear that he might be killed. . . . The point I am making is the inappropriateness of his making so much of the little notice on the cigarette package, smoking may be harmful, which he would obey, and yet feeling that this other thing was real. I think it is inconsistent with that of a mentally stable mind.

I tried to turn Humme's testimony around by asking if he thought it would be "inappropriate" for Wright "to fear one type of injury to his body (threats) and not fear another (smoking)." Remembering that Humme thought it was inappropriate for Jerome to believe threats communicated to him by other prisoners, inappropriate for him to believe he would not be fearful outside the prison, and inappropriate for him to be concerned about physical injury and lung cancer at the same time, I was astonished by his answer: "I don't think appropriateness is the point here." That was my first introduction to the flexible language of psychiatry. Later, I would learn that the phrase "inappropriate affect" crops up in almost every commitment report. That, and the phrase "insight nil," which means "I think this person is crazy but he disagrees," have been the principal grounds for commitment in almost every case I have ever handled.

Dorsey then called Dr. Max Dahl, assistant director of Hudson River State Hospital. Dahl had examined Jerome Wright with Humme, and he too had concluded that Wright was "acutely mentally ill, suffering from paranoid schizophrenia." On cross-examination, Dahl testified that he was "in substantial agreement" with the testimony of his colleague.

Q. Doctor, in your evaluation, would it be relevant if I stated to you that I intended to introduce as witnesses other prisoners who will testify that they have themselves told Jerome Wright that his life is, in fact, in danger? Would that be relevant to your examination?

A. No, it would not influence my opinion. I would say that this is one of those mental cases where statements made by a patient are proven to be true, but the reactions of the patient to these statements are so absurd that they can only be tied in with mental illness.

Q. Doctor, if these statements that his life was in danger were, in fact, proven to be true, and those statements had been communicated to him, which of his responses to those statements would have been inappropriate?

A. Well, it would be inappropriate, first of all, that he believes them.

Finally, Dorsey called Dr. Stephen Petres. Certain that Humme and Dahl would say Wright was mentally ill, I had earlier asked the court to appoint an independent psychiatrist (the clerk keeps a list of those available for such a purpose)—hence, Dr. Petres. It turned out, however, that Petres also worked at Hudson River State Hospital—as a "staff member." It was not likely he would disagree with his superiors, and he didn't.

Q. Doctor, would it be a relevant consideration in your examination if at least one other prisoner had told Mr. Wright that it was a matter of general knowledge in the prison population that his life was in danger? Would that influence your decision as to whether or not some of his statements and behavior would be symptomatic of mental illness?

A. No . . . because he accepted the prisoner's statement that he might be killed. . . . He accepted the delusions as a fact, so on that he has not any insight and he clearly shows the presence of a very dangerous delusion.

Q. In other words, you are testifying that his acceptance of these statements as fact is an indication that he is mentally ill?

A. Well, yes.

The state rested, and while the court reporter changed his tapes, I began quickly to rough out a defense. If Jerome Wright was crazy, so was Warden Follette, who had believed Wright's concern for his safety warranted special protective measures, at added cost and inconvenience to the state, including placing Wright in a segregated security cell for almost a year. And the prison psychiatrist who had examined Wright while he was in the security cell had not considered his fears unreasonable. He had recommended parole and had reported to the Commutation Board that he found no evidence of psychosis or mental illness. Indeed, although Doctors Humme, Dahl, and Petres all said they had read the prison file, they had somehow failed to note that prior to December 4, 1968, the day he wrote the crucial letter, Jerome had been examined by at least four different psychiatrists, all of whom had concluded that he was not mentally ill or psychotic. But I wasn't sure that would be enough, so I asked Judge Joseph F. Hawkins for a brief recess.

Jerome Wright and I huddled at the end of the hall. Never the first to speak, he waited quietly as I skimmed through my notes. "Mr. Wright, you can see from the testimony that the doctors think you're crazy because you believe your life is in danger and they don't. If other prisoners testify that your life *is* in danger, that would go a long way toward proving them wrong. I want you to reconsider giving me their names."

"I can't do it."

"Why not?"

"Because then they'd get me for sure."

"Just one name will do. It doesn't even have to be someone who threatened you, just someone who knows about it."

Finally, in a voice weary with resignation, he muttered, "Ezra Martin."

"Who?"

"Ezra Martin. He knows about it. He's one of the ones who warned me about it."

"Will he testify?"

"I don't know."

Ten minutes later, Ezra Martin was led up the interior metal staircase, a guard on either side. We conversed alone.

"Do you know what this is all about?"

"No."

"Well, I'm a lawyer. I represent Mr. Jerome Wright. Do you know him?"

"Yes."

"When was the last time you talked to him?"

"About a month ago."

"Mr. Wright told me that you could give me some idea of his reputation among the other prisoners. Is that right?"

"What do you mean?"

My answer was evasive because I did not want to lead him; I wanted to learn for myself if Jerome was telling the truth. "Well, you know. Just general stuff. Did they like him or not? Did he have a lot of friends?"

"I don't think he had many friends. He kept pretty much to himself. Besides, he was in segregation."

"Why was that?"

"Because he was supposed to be an informer."

"What do you mean?"

"Well, I heard he was supposed to be an informer and that's why he was in segregation, for his own good."

When I was reasonably sure Martin was telling the truth, I headed back to the courtroom and called as my first witness Jerome Wright, who testified that other prisoners had told him he was considered to be an informer and that his safety was therefore in danger.

Dorsey's cross-examination did not change Wright's story, but it did inadvertently reveal a common danger of psychiatric interviews—the leading question. One of the doctors had told Dorsey that Wright thought he might be "poisoned," and, as his last question, Dorsey asked Wright about that.

Q. Did you tell any of those doctors that you were afraid that somebody was going to "put poison in my food"?

A. No. One doctor asked me what did I think, had I said something about my food being poisoned. I said, "No." He said, "Well, if they are trying to kill you, they could poison your food." I said, "Yes, that's possible."

Ezra Martin was next.

Q. Mr. Martin, what, if any, statements have you heard concerning Mr. Wright?
A. I had heard as to the fact that the inmate, Jerome Wright, was considered an informer, and due to that, that he was placed in segregation for protection for his own good.

There was more. Martin testified about his "conversations" with Wright. Jerome's mother testified that there were a home and a job waiting for him, and that he had absolutely no history of hospitalization or treatment for mental illness.

Then it was time for the legal arguments I had thought would be the only issue in the case. Dorsey conceded that but for the one letter Wright would have been paroled. After a brief discussion of the constitutional points and the cases which supported them, I handed the judge my fourteen-page brief and rested. I expected him to reserve judgment until he had read my brief and thought over the three hours of testimony, but I was wrong. Before I could return to my chair, Judge Hawkins announced his decision.

THE COURT: All right, this Court has held a hearing according to the Order of Mr. Justice Supple upon the alleged mental illness of one Jerome Wright. It is the decision of this Court that the said Jerome Wright, based upon the medical evidence received and educed before this Court, is mentally ill and it is proper that he be forwarded to the Dannemora Institution for Treatment of Mental Disease. The Order is signed as of this date.

I was stunned. Wright's was my first trial (Youngblood's would be the second), and I had not believed until then that a man could be labeled mad without substantially more proof than the court had heard, or that a judge would cavalierly dismiss constitutional objections, which I knew from my research were substantial, without so much as a glance at the brief.

Wright stood quietly in the corridor, tears in his eyes, as his mother, straining to be cheerful, talked about an appeal. "No, Mother, it's no use. I'll never see you again. They'll get me now for sure." Two guards led him down the stairs and out of sight. I could say nothing to the Wrights. They had known, better than I, that Jerome would not win. Nonetheless, discouraged as they were, they asked me to appeal.

Perfecting an appeal, as it is called, is not as simple as the layman might suppose. The rules are many, and they vary from court to court. I worked my way through the rules and came up with a forty-page appellate brief. Underlying the constitutional arguments I would make on appeal was a very simple point that had nothing to do with the law. If Jerome was, in fact, paranoid, it was clear that he was afraid only of other prisoners—on the outside he would "sit around, take a drink, and laugh about it." Surely the best way to treat his paranoia, if such it was, would be to set him free. Instead, the state proposed to cancel his parole and confine him for two more years among a host of prisoners, any one of whom, in Jerome's view, might kill him.

My brief raised three points of law. First, the factual finding that Jerome was paranoid was not supported by substantial evidence. The only evidence of mental illness was the opinion of Doctors Humme, Dahl, and Petres. Generally, a court will receive as evidence only facts, not opinion. But there is an exception for doctors and other "expert" witnesses; unlike the average witness, experts are permitted to give opinions. Still, I had found an exception to the exception—several courts had ruled that opinion testimony was valueless if the opinion was based upon an assumed state of facts unless the assumption was later proved to be true. The three doctors had found Jerome paranoid because of their assumption that his life was not, in fact, in danger—an assumption that neither they nor the state ever sought to prove.

Second, since the question to be determined—was Wright mentally ill?—was *exactly* the same question as was involved in civil commitment proceedings, it should have been decided by the same procedures afforded nonprisoners, including the right to a jury trial, which Wright did not have. To offer less would constitute an unreasonable classification in violation of the "equal protection" clause of the Fourteenth Amendment to the United States Constitution, which requires that all persons be given the same legal protections unless there is a very good reason for treating them differently.

Third, because there was no penal justification for further confinement (Wright had been slated for parole), he should be hospitalized, if at all, in a civil mental hospital, not Dannemora. Courts had already ruled that a prisoner who became mentally ill just as his sentence was about to expire, or after he had actually been released on parole, must be treated in a civil hospital, and there was no reasonable basis for treating Wright differently.

On April 24, 1969, the day before the state's answering brief was due, Tom Dorsey called to tell me that Wright had been discharged from Dannemora as "not mentally ill" and had immediately been released on parole. And so, said Dorsey, the appeal was moot. In other words, since Wright had been granted the relief he was seeking, there was nothing for the appellate court to decide and no reason to pursue the appeal.

Jerome Wright's case taught me that judges will usually accept the unchallenged opinions of psychiatrists, no matter how weak they seem, and that a prospective patient cannot win a factual hearing without expert testimony on his side. More important, I now knew that the state has a weapon in its test-case arsenal that the private litigant cannot match. When faced with a difficult issue and a good chance it will lose, the state can simply let the patient go, claim the case is moot, and continue with its policies, unhampered by adverse precedent. (That is exactly what happened in four of my next five cases, and almost happened in von Wolfersdorf's.) Equally important, the state can select the cases it will allow to proceed to decision, thereby ensuring that legal issues, when they reach the court, come wrapped in the factual situations most favorable to the state.

The Wright case also taught me to distrust the expertise of psychiatrists. Later, I would learn that psychiatrists disagree with each other—more, in fact, than do experts from any other discipline—almost as often as they agree, and that psychiatry remains an imprecise discipline relying heavily on subjective judgment. I would also learn that whether a person is labeled mentally ill depends very little on his mental condition and a great deal on the personal—not the medical or scientific—beliefs and values of the particular psychiatrist who examines him.

Postscript

The state let Jerome Wright go, but it kept Roy Schuster, also a client of my office, whose case had been filed before I was hired. Like Wright, Schuster had been transferred from prison to Dannemora without a jury trial. But Schuster, unlike Wright, had been convicted of a crime of violence (second-degree murder of his wife), and the state was not about to make his case moot by letting him go.

Shortly after Wright was released, a federal appeals court ruled that Schuster and all the other Dannemora inmates were constitutionally entitled to receive "substantially all the procedures granted to noncriminals who are involuntarily committed as patients in civil mental hospitals," including the right to a jury trial on the issue of their mental health. They would not be released if they won the jury trial, but they would be retransferred out of Dannemora and back to prison. Within the month, 80 per cent of the Dannemora inmates had requested jury trials, asking, in effect, to be sent to prison.

Part II
Behind Locked Doors

Good intentions will always be pleaded for every assumption of power. . . . It is hardly too strong to say that the Constitution was made to guard the public against the dangers of good intentions. There are men in all ages, and supporting all causes, who mean to govern well, but they mean to govern. They promise to be good masters, but they mean to be masters.

—DANIEL WEBSTER

If pressed, mental hospital administrators will admit that 95 per cent of their patients are not dangerous; they are hospitalized because, though harmless, they are mentally ill and need treatment.

Whether they "need" treatment or not, they do not get it, unless treatment can be defined as manual labor eight hours a day, six days a week.

These next four chapters are about life inside the hospital. The stories are very different; but, in a way, they are alike. Each one is about the enormous disparity between what mental hospitals are supposed to be and what they really are. They are supposed to be places where troubled people receive care and attention from a gentle and dedicated staff. They are, instead, places where sick people get sicker and sane people go mad, where the hours are filled not with compassion, but with neglect.

5 / Warehouse I

And when he is out of sight, quickly also is he out of mind.
—THOMAS A KEMPIS
Imitation of Christ
Book I, Chapter 23

In 1834, it was an arsenal, stockpiling weapons for defense against Seminole Indian raids. In 1877, the weapons were replaced by patients and the name was changed to "asylum," but the Florida State Hospital remained a warehouse; only the inventory changed. By 1957, the "hospital," located just outside Chattahoochee, Florida, near the Georgia and Alabama borders, housed 5,000 patients. It was run-down, understaffed, and overcrowded. For almost fifty years the patient population had exceeded the hospital's authorized capacity. One of the patients was Kenneth Donaldson, listed in the inventory as No. A-25738.

In August of 1956, Donaldson, a forty-eight-year-old divorced Philadelphia carpenter, had traveled south to the Bellair Village Trailer Court, in Pinellas County, Florida, for an extended visit with his eighty-year-old parents. The visit, their first in many years, was pleasant, and nothing unusual happened for several months. Then, in late November, Donaldson began to feel drowsy, and he mentioned to his father that someone, perhaps one of the neighbors, might be putting something in his food. When asked why he even suspected such an unlikely thing, Donaldson told his parents of a similar episode that had happened to him three years earlier, while he was living in Lynnwood, California, a suburb of Los Angeles. Donaldson had eaten regularly in the same Lynnwood diner. One day, shortly after lunch, he began to feel peculiar, and he went to a physician recommended by his landlady. The physician took a urine sample and sent it to a laboratory. The lab report, which Donaldson still has, confirmed the presence of a large amount of codeine, a sedative, in his urine. Donaldson had not been taking any cough syrup, which sometimes contains codeine, or any other medication (he was a follower of the Christian Science faith), so he reasoned that the codeine must have been placed in his food, either on purpose or by accident. He never ate at the diner again and had no recurrence of the drowsiness until the Florida episode.

On December 10, Donaldson's father filed with the Pinellas County Court a petition requesting a sanity hearing for his son, claiming that because of "persecution complex, [and] increasing signs of paranoid delusions, petitioner believes him to be potentially dangerous." Later that day, police officers arrested Donaldson and took him to the Pinellas County jail in Clearwater. On the thirteenth, Jack F. White, the county judge, ordered the sheriff of Pinellas County to summon an "examining committee." Two of the committee members, J. O. Norton and Virgil D. Smith, were physicians, but not psychiatrists. The third, Wilmer James, was the Pinellas County deputy sheriff. Later that day, each of the three committee members signed a printed form stating that the committee had made "a thorough examination" of Donaldson's "mental and physical condition." Most of the form was left blank. The committee added only Donaldson's age and, at the bottom of the printed form, that he suffered from "paranoid schizophrenia," that his particular hallucinations were "auditory" and "visual," and that his propensities were "delusions."

These five words, inserted in a form, would serve as the basis for Donaldson's commitment. More troubling than the sketchiness of the report was Donaldson's claim that he was not actually seen by the committee members until several days after they had signed the form. Donaldson kept a detailed diary of that period, so that many years later he was able to describe the circumstances of his jailhouse examination.

A. I had been locked up some weeks about the middle of my stay there, the stay was five weeks altogether, and the nurse came along one morning and said, "The doctor is coming. Get ready." I was dressed anyway. So in a couple of minutes the doctor came and said, "Hello." I said, "Hello." I said, "I don't need a doctor. I need a lawyer." "Oh, you do, huh?" You know, you'd think I was a smart aleck. And he asked me questions about what day it was, did I know where I was, and I believe he said, "Is it raining outside?" That's all. And he walked out. Possibly the last week I was there, or close to it, a man in the second cell down had a heart attack during the night. The doctor didn't come until breakfast time and after the doctor had taken care of him, ordered him out to the hospital, then the doctor stopped by and just said, "Hello," and he asked the same as this other doctor did. That was my examination.

Q. Approximately how long did you speak with each doctor?

A. Less than two minutes with each doctor.

Eventually, said Donaldson, Judge White came to his cell and told him that because the doctors had found him to be in need of hospitalization, he would be sent to Florida State Hospital, in the northwest corner of the state. Donaldson, however, demanded a judicial hearing, and as the judge walked away, he shouted that he wanted a lawyer, too. The judge came back and promised to send a lawyer. On January 3, 1957, a lawyer arrived and told Donaldson that his fee would be $35 (which he never collected), the amount Donaldson happened to have in his billfold at the sheriff's desk. The lawyer left and came back a few minutes later to report that the doctors could not attend a hearing for at least two more weeks. Donaldson said, "All right. What's the difference? I'll wait two more weeks." The lawyer said, "No, we'll have the hearing right away, and if we need another hearing later, we'll have it later." Donaldson agreed, but told the lawyer he wouldn't get a cent until the doctors appeared in court.

Donaldson was then led downstairs to the visitors' room and locked in the wire prisoners' cage. Judge White came in, followed by the lawyer, and sat behind a desk facing Donaldson. No one else was present. Donaldson told the judge that he wanted the doctors there "in person to tell me why I was crazy," but the judge ignored that request and asked Donaldson to tell his story. Donaldson had said only a few words about his past life when the lawyer left the room, never to return. He had not said a single word. After Donaldson had talked a few minutes longer, the judge rose and told him that he would be sent to Florida State Hospital for a few weeks of "rest." Thereupon the judge signed another printed form, this one titled "Order Adjudging Incompetency." The order recited, verbatim, the report of the examining committee. Eight days later, Donaldson was transferred to Florida State Hospital, where he would be held for fifteen years without ever again appearing before a judge.

Only rarely during his first four years did a doctor or nurse so much as pass through Donaldson's ward. Doctors were seen in their offices, by invitation only. One or two such contacts per year were considered better than average. It was not uncommon for patients to go two, three, or even four years without speaking to a doctor. Life on the wards was governed by untrained and occasionally brutal attendants who were drawn from the two surrounding counties—counties that had the highest level of functional illiteracy in the nation; many of the attendants could neither read nor write.

Donaldson's ward doctor was almost totally occupied in preparing court papers for the 350 patients in Donaldson's section who had been charged with or convicted of crimes, most of whom still faced a trial, a sentencing hearing, or an appeal. But for Donaldson and the other civil patients—those not charged with any crime—the judicial process was over. Their commitments were by law "indefinite," and thus lacked the urgency of the criminal commitments.

Intelligent and articulate, Donaldson rapidly became the "scribe" and spokesman for his section. In 1961, largely because of his documented complaints to public officials, the Florida legislature established a committee to investigate the hospital. The committee report described Donaldson's building as "antiquated," "completely obsolete," and "a serious fire hazard." The wards were "maintained more as detention wards for inmates than as hospital wards for the sick." It was a "common practice" for attendants to "choke" agitated patients until they were subdued. The committee discovered "strip cells," where patients were held naked in solitary confinement, without bedding or exercise, for "prolonged" periods. Attendants, not doctors, decided which patients would be put there and for how long. A "large number" of those attendants had "less than a high school education" and were "ill-equipped for the responsible care and treatment of patients." The average take-home pay for attendants was less than $1,700 per year. Forced to moonlight in order to survive, the attendants frequently were too exhausted to give patients the attention they required and considered their duties "almost exclusively custodial in nature."

The hospital, in general, was "extremely short of doctors," the report continued, but the shortage was most acute in Donaldson's section, where "during 1960 and prior to that time, there was only one doctor [an obstetrician] responsible for the care and treatment of approximately 1,000 [male] patients" (the American Psychiatric Association considered one doctor for every 150 patients to be the absolute minimum). There was no psychiatrist, no psychologist, and, except in the infirmary, no nurse. At 5:00 P.M. (and, presumably, on weekends), the nurse and the obstetrician went home. Patients who developed physical ailments during the night were out of luck. Most depressing of all, the committee found that "a number of patients are well or may be curable, but the doctors are reluctant to spend much time with them because there is little or no chance of their being discharged because there is no one in society to accept responsibility for them."

One of those patients was Kenneth Donaldson. The obstetrician had told Donaldson he could be discharged if his father would accept custody; but his father would not.

The committee report troubled the Florida legislature, though not sufficiently to pry loose the money for hiring enough doctors, psychologists, nurses, and social workers so that Florida State Hospital could be converted from a warehouse to a treatment facility. The executive branch eventually requested money to fund 159 new positions, but the legislature refused to fund even one.

After the report, years went by and nothing changed. The Joint Commission on the Accreditation of Hospitals, an agency sponsored by the American Medical Association and several other professional organizations, refused to accredit Florida State, finding it unworthy of the name "hospital" (one-third of the mental hospitals in the United States are not accredited). The legislature was unmoved. Other studies followed. In 1963, the American Psychiatric Association recommended more personnel for Florida State. In 1970, the Florida Medical Association concurred, finding that the budget was sufficient only "for a custodial-type mental health program" and that "psychiatric care," usually by a "foreign-born or trained doctor not yet licensed in Florida," was "modest and not as intensive as would be desired." Still the legislature did nothing.

Kenneth Donaldson knew the legislature could not be shaken from its indifference. He expected better from the courts, but he was wrong. Eighteen times in fifteen years, Donaldson tried to interest courts in his plight, always without success. His argument was threefold: (1) At his commitment hearing, he had not actually been represented by counsel and had had no opportunity to cross-examine the examining committee. (2) He was not then, and was not now, mentally ill or dangerous. (3) Most important, even if he *was* to some degree mentally ill, the state had withheld from him the psychiatric treatment necessary for a cure.

The third point asserted a new right, the "right to treatment," first articulated in 1960 by Morton Birnbaum, who was both an M.D. (though not a psychiatrist) and a lawyer. Birnbaum's analysis was simple but compelling: if the patient is confined not because he is considered dangerous, but because of a supposed need for treatment, then, failing such treatment, the justification for confinement disappears. No one thought Donaldson was dangerous; neither before nor during his fifteen years of hospitalization did he commit or even threaten a violent act. The state said he was there because he needed treatment, but he got none. He had received no individual or group psychotherapy and rarely had he seen a doctor. Except for one two-week period, he had not even received psychiatric medication.

Time after time Donaldson made these allegations and begged the courts for an opportunity to prove them. Always the courts said no. Typical was the decision of County Court Judge H. Y. Reynolds in rejecting Donaldson's 1968 request for a habeas corpus hearing: "Certainly the State Hospital Authorities have no desire nor reason to detain you in the hospital any longer than your condition requires. In the event your condition is such as to justify it, the medical staff will give you a hearing." (The staff had given Donaldson three hearings—one in 1962, five years after he was hospitalized, one in 1964, and one in 1968.)

The courts in effect said hands off, thereby abandoning Donaldson and thousands like him to the unreviewable opinions of the very men whose judgment Donaldson was contesting. The state of Florida never denied any of Donaldson's allegations. The courts, both state and federal, simply refused, again and again, to let him stand before a judge and tell his story.

Four times Donaldson's appeal reached the United States Supreme Court, only to be denied. The fourth time, however, the Supreme Court took the unusual step of stating that its denial of Donaldson's petition was "without prejudice" to his "right to apply to the appropriate United States District Court for relief." The wording suggested that the nine justices of the Supreme Court were finally interested in the constitutional issues raised by confinement without treatment, but were not ready to resolve those legal issues until after the factual allegations of inadequate treatment had been proved at trial.

To Morton Birnbaum, who for five years had been serving without fee as Donaldson's lawyer (before then, Donaldson had drafted his own court papers), this meant that after fifteen years Donaldson might receive a judicial hearing on his claims.

In connection with Donaldson's fourth petition to the Supreme Court, I had written an *amicus curiae*, or friend-of-the-court, brief on behalf of the American Civil Liberties Union, urging the Court to consider Donaldson's plea, and Birnbaum asked if I would now join him as cocounsel. Together we drafted a combined habeas corpus petition and civil rights act complaint, which requested Donaldson's release and $100,000 damages for the fifteen years he had been held without treatment. We brought suit as a "class action" on behalf of Donaldson and all the other patients in Florida State Hospital. That was February 24, 1971. On March 10, Federal Judge David L. Middlebrooks, who sits in Tallahassee, forty miles from the hospital, dismissed the complaint. We requested reargument and on April 26, under our prodding, he reversed himself and ruled that Donaldson was entitled to a hearing. Nevertheless, on his own initiative, he transferred the case to Judge Joseph Lieb, in Tampa, 270 miles to the south, for further proceedings.

Birnbaum and I then made a trip to Tampa. Judge Lieb could see no reason for the case to be before him, and neither could we, so he sent it back to Judge Middlebrooks. Eventually, after more skirmishing, Judge Middlebrooks scheduled a pretrial conference to be held on August 12, 1971. Faced with the prospect of having at last to justify their actions to a federal judge, the hospital officials moved fast. On July 31, less than two weeks before the pretrial conference, the hospital director certified that Donaldson, after fifteen years of hopeless insanity, had suddenly recovered and was "no longer incompetent." Donaldson was discharged and placed on a bus for Tallahassee. The state attorney general then made a motion to dismiss Donaldson's complaint, arguing that since he had been discharged, his case was moot.

On the twelfth, Birnbaum and I flew to Tallahassee and met Donaldson for breakfast in the L & T Café. He seemed younger than his sixty-three years. His face was creased, but handsome in a rugged, outdoors way. He was quiet, as if he were constantly thinking of serious matters, and reserved, though not at all somber. In fact, he was enthusiastic and quick to laugh. I noticed he was wearing new shoes. He chuckled and said that the first thing he had done in Tallahassee, after finding a rooming house, was to buy a sport shirt, an umbrella, and two pairs of shoes. For the past twelve days he had risen early and walked until dark, exploring every corner of Tallahassee, learning again what it meant to be free. At night he read or went to a movie.

We walked to the courthouse, three blocks away, and were soon sitting in Judge Middlebrooks's chambers. The hearing was informal, almost like a round-table discussion, though argument was heated. The judge indicated that he was going to dismiss Donaldson's complaint on somewhat technical grounds. He would, however, give us ten days to file an amended complaint, which through slightly different wording could avoid those technical objections. He ruled that Donaldson's discharge from the hospital did not make moot his own claim for damages, as the defendants had argued; but he agreed with the defendants that, because of his discharge, Donaldson was no longer a bona fide representative of the patients still in the hospital. For that reason, the case could not, as we had hoped, proceed as a class action. Still, it had been held, for the first time in the United States, that an involuntary patient can sue for money damages if he is not given adequate treatment.

The pretrial hearing ended about noon. Dr. Birnbaum and I left immediately for Florida State Hospital for our first look at Donaldson's hospital record, which Judge Middlebrooks had ruled we had a right to inspect. The record consisted of three small folders, two of which contained nothing but correspondence to, from, and about Donaldson. The third, the "medical folder," required only sixty-three pages to describe Donaldson's fifteen years as a mental patient, and many of the pages were just forms or summaries of previous pages. Comments by doctors were called "Progress Notes." The progress notes describing Donaldson's first ten years at Florida State filled only six pages.

The medical folder, though skimpy, contained much we had not known before, and much that corroborated Donaldson's allegations. Most of the progress notes simply stated in a sentence or two that Donaldson ate and slept well, was quiet and co-operative, but refused to admit he was mentally ill. Many of them concluded with a recommendation to "continue custodial care." Nowhere could we find a treatment program, or any indication of what the hospital proposed to do for Donaldson, other than feed and clothe him. There seemed to be general agreement that Donaldson was not at all dangerous to himself or to others. But he persisted in believing that someone had put codeine in his food and that he was not a resident of Florida.* The complete progress note for April 3, 1962, said: "Resides on ward #8, shows no particular change mentally, he is still delusional and paranoid with impaired judgment. He has no other object in his life than his transfer to New Jersey State. Still persists he is a New Jersey resident and refuses to submit to injustice. Continue custodial care." The note for August 30, 1965: "Physically no complaints. He states he feels physically well. Mentally he maintains the idea that he is all right now and doesn't belong here. Continue custodial care." Those notes are representative of the others.

Except for a few hours with a psychiatrist during his first two weeks at the hospital, there was no indication in the medical folder that any doctor had spent more than five or ten minutes talking with Donaldson until 1968, when a doctor named Israel Hanenson, since deceased, took an interest in his case and tried unsuccessfully to get him discharged. On April 30, 1969, Dr. Hanenson wrote: "At the present time it is the opinion of this examiner that this patient is most definitely in remission of his past psychiatric symptoms and has been so for some time." Yet Donaldson was held at Florida State for more than two more years.

In 1962, more than five years after his commitment, Donald-

---

* Under Florida law, no one could legally be hospitalized at Florida State Hospital unless he had been a resident of the state for one year prior to hospitalization. The examining committee had reported Donaldson as living with his parents in Florida for four years when, in fact, he had been there only four months. Before that, he had lived in Camden, New Jersey. But because he continued to deny that he was, as the examining committee reported, a resident of Florida, the hospital decided he was paranoid and had impaired judgment.

son received his first staff hearing—a review of his case before a panel of hospital doctors. Three of the doctors at that hearing recommended that Donaldson be given some "intensive treatment and medication," but nothing came of their recommendation. In January of 1964, because a member of the Florida Senate intervened in Donaldson's behalf, he was again presented to the staff. Once again, nothing changed.

Between 1964 and 1968, John Lembecke, an old college friend of Donaldson's (he had attended Syracuse University for a year and a half), tried numerous times to persuade the hospital to release Donaldson to his custody. Lembecke was a certified public accountant, and lived with his wife and children in Binghamton, New York. He wrote and visited the hospital several times, promising to provide for Donaldson's room and board and to accept responsibility for his conduct. After years of pressure, a third staff hearing was convened, in March of 1968, and unanimously recommended to Dr. J. B. O'Connor, then director of Florida State, that Donaldson be released to Lembecke on an out-of-state discharge.

O'Connor, however, told Lembecke that he could not release Donaldson until Lembecke had obtained the written, notarized consent of Donaldson's ninety-year-old parents. Lembecke did so. At the last moment, with the necessary consent in hand, O'Connor changed his mind and refused to follow the staff recommendation.

There was no conceivable reason for denying Lembecke's request. But O'Connor apparently needed no reason. He was content to dismiss the request on the ground that Lembecke, too, must be crazy. Across the top of one of Lembecke's letters, O'Connor had casually jotted a note to a Dr. Gumanis, the physician in charge of Donaldson's section: "This man, himself, must not be well to want to get involved with someone like this patient. . . . Recommend turn it down."

There was no way to win O'Connor's game. For years Donaldson had been confined because there was "no one to take care of him" on the outside. Then, when a reputable outsider offered to take care of him, the offer was rejected. Earlier, Helping Hands, Incorporated, a halfway house that provided homes and jobs for former mental patients, had offered, in response to Donaldson's request, to receive and supervise him as one of its six residents. O'Connor had squelched that offer, too, claiming that if released, Donaldson would "require very strict supervision which he would not tolerate."

The hospital record also showed clearly that Donaldson had received no psychiatric medication, no group therapy, nothing worthy of the name "treatment."

The next day, the hospital's lawyers took Donaldson's deposition—his answers, under oath, to their questions—and we took the deposition of Dr. Francis G. Walls, who had recently been the acting superintendent of Florida State Hospital and who, with O'Connor and other hospital officials, was named as a defendant in the case.

Walls admitted the truth of much of what Donaldson had been claiming for years. In his deposition, he conceded that Donaldson had not been considered by him or anyone else at the hospital to be physically dangerous to himself or to others. He admitted that at Florida State there were only twenty-eight physicians for 5,000 patients, and that only eight of those physicians were licensed to practice medicine in Florida. And he confessed much more: there were only eighteen psychiatrists, of whom four were licensed to practice medicine and only two were board-certified; as late as March, 1970, there was only one psychiatrist to treat the 800 patients in the area of the hospital where Donaldson was confined; and the eighteen psychiatrists spent approximately 50 per cent of their time performing administrative and other nonpsychiatric functions—in effect, there was only one *clinical* psychiatrist for every 625 patients. The "ideal," said Walls, "is one psychiatrist for every [50] acutely ill persons and one for every 125 chronically ill persons," and he allowed that even in a "practical" situation—one that was far less than ideal—Florida State should have had "another twenty psychiatrists and ten or more physicians," which would have been "just about double" its staff at the time. He then conceded that the number of "nurses" at Florida State was also "inadequate at the present time," with the hospital in need of "about another forty" nurses; that existing treatment programs were "not what they should be"; and that "we haven't sufficient staff—we could do a better job with more staff. It's really a matter of numbers, you see." Finally, he admitted that the hospital did not have an "individualized treatment program" for Donaldson and that the hospital records did not specify any treatment goals or plans for him. Nevertheless, even though he did not think Donaldson was dangerous, and even though he thought Donaldson's chances for recovery were very poor, Dr. Walls testified that if he had been in charge, he would have kept Donaldson in the hospital for the rest of his life. Why? "Because he is mentally ill."

During his own deposition, Donaldson calmly detailed his years of boredom and neglect. He began by describing a typical interview with a doctor.

A. The doctor has a three-by-five file card on his desk and the patient's name on each card, and each time you go see him, he fills in one line. He had three questions at that time. He invariably asked each patient, "What ward are you on? Are you taking any medication? Are you working anyplace?" You answered those three questions. "That'll be all." When I'd first go in for the interview [he would say], "I have a letter from so and so. Do you know this person?" I'd say, "Yes." Then he'd ask me the three questions. "That'll be all."
   . . .
   And one day I complained about not getting any therapy of any kind and the doctor pulled out his three-by-five card, read off

each date, and he said, "That is psychotherapy. You have been getting psychotherapy."

Q. What did you say to him at that time? Did you make any response to that statement?

A. Yes, I did. I didn't swear, but I should have.

Q. Mr. Donaldson, let me ask you, are you saying that that was the typical encounter with a doctor?

A. It was almost the only encounter anyone had with the doctor.

Q. Did you ever sit down and engage in an extensive discussion with any psychiatrist about your past, or your mental condition, or any plans for your future?

A. The first day at the receiving ward, Dr. Adair, I don't know whether it's C. H., something like that.

Q. Any time since then other than staff conferences?

A. Since then, yes, sir. Possibly the first couple of times or so I talked to Dr. O'Conner, I talked for five minutes or so; and Dr. Gumanis talked to me for maybe five or ten minutes, or maybe five minutes a couple of times in all the years I knew him. When I got over to C Department, Dr. Hanenson spent a lot of time with me.

Q. When was that, please?

A. I got over there April 18, 1967, and Dr. Hanenson spent more time with me in the first year that I was in C Department than all the other doctors in the hospital had in the ten years up until then.

Q. Is it accurate to say, Mr. Donaldson, that except for your initial admission interview by Dr. Adair, that in the entire period of your hospitalization, between that time and your interviews with Dr. Hanenson, you did not speak with any psychiatrist for more than five minutes or so at a time?

A. That's right, and usually it would be less than two minutes.

Q. And is it also correct that usually it would involve those three typical questions and that is all?

A. That is right.

After the depositions, Donaldson, Birnbaum, and I had dinner in the Tallahassee Airport restaurant. We were pleased with what we had learned in our first two days of preparation for trial, but we knew that our case, no matter how strong, was probably lost. Florida State Hospital was one of the largest employers in the area, and several of the jurors would probably be relatives of persons who depended for their living on continued employment at Florida State. Such jurors were not likely to be sympathetic to a lawsuit that challenged the adequacy of treatment in "their" hospital and requested money damages from Dr. O'Connor, an important man in their community. If O'Connor testified, we could probably force him to admit the truth of many of our allegations. He had already refused to testify, however, claiming his heart could not stand the strain. Unless the court ordered O'Connor to testify—and that was unlikely—it would be difficult to prove important parts of our claim.

Still, there was a fighting chance that Donaldson would recover at least some financial compensation for the years he had been held without treatment. Although the trial would not be held for several months, there was plenty to do—questioning other hospital employees, rounding up expert witnesses to testify on Donaldson's behalf, and so on. For now, however, we could relax. With obvious delight, Donaldson turned to the waitress and asked her to bring him a cold bottle of beer, the first he had ordered in fifteen years.

After dinner, Birnbaum and I flew back to New York City and Donaldson took the bus to Syracuse, New York. Three days later, he found an apartment and a job as a hotel clerk and night auditor, a job he has held without incident ever since.

6 / Warehouse II

That Florida State Hospital is a human warehouse does not make it unique. Hundreds like it can be found all over the country. One of them, Bryce State Hospital, is located in Tuscaloosa, Alabama. It was built by slave labor during the Civil War, and its wide, white-columned porch and sweeping lawn dominated by an ancient pistachio tree give Bryce the graceful look of a southern mansion. Behind the façade, however, treatment is nonexistent. Excluding the administrative staff, there were until recently only two full-time psychiatrists to supervise the 5,000 patients, and only one psychologist with a Ph.D. degree. The wards are filled with human misery.

I first learned of Bryce on January 10, 1971, when I received a long-distance call from George Dean, one of the South's most colorful—and capable—lawyers. Almost by accident, he had stumbled onto a major right-to-treatment case, which at the time was limited to Bryce but would soon encompass the patients in every mental institution in Alabama. I knew immediately that the case would have nationwide impact because the judge, Frank Johnson, Jr., was one of the three or four most respected federal district court judges in the nation.

Dean knew about the Donaldson case. He was calling because he needed to become overnight an expert on the right to treatment. I described the major cases and authorities over the telephone. That night I assembled a more extensive set of materials and sent them to Dean by special delivery. Except for two more telephone calls requesting additional information, Dean took it from there. By March 11, he had convinced Judge Johnson that involuntary mental patients did have a *constitutional* right to adequate treatment. That was important, because only a handful of judges had accepted the right-to-treatment argument. But Judge Johnson had gone one step further. Ruling that the patients at Bryce State Hospital were not, in fact, receiving adequate treatment, he had given the defendants—all were officials or agencies of the state of Alabama—six months to provide adequate treatment, indicating that if they failed, he would either release the patients or appoint a panel of experts to run the hospital.

In two months George Dean had accomplished what other lawyers had been attempting for years. But the case was now too big for one lawyer and Dean needed help. Up to this point, the case had been relatively uncomplicated. Judge Johnson had not found it necessary to fix standards against which the adequacy of treatment at Bryce could be measured, because the patients at Bryce received *no* treatment. Most of them had no contact at all with psychiatrists or psychologists, and that was clearly inadequate treatment. But what if a psychiatrist talked with each patient once a week, or once a month? Would that be adequate?

There were literally hundreds of such questions. Bryce spent fifty cents per day per patient for food. Was that enough to provide an adequate diet? If not, how much did a nutritious diet cost? No one would deny that adequate treatment could be provided only in a humane physical environment. Did that mean the state was constitutionally obligated to install air conditioning in the oppressive back wards, where old people died of dehydration in the Alabama summers? Everyone would agree that a treatment program should give patients a sense of dignity. Did that give patients the right to wear their own clothes, to send and receive uncensored mail, to make and receive telephone calls? And exactly how much space should be required per patient? When should a hospital be considered overcrowded? How frequently must the hospital review each patient's progress? Was there a maximum length of time beyond which hospitalization became antitherapeutic?

These and similar questions had to be answered, both in order to evaluate the state's progress at the end of the six months granted by Judge Johnson and to provide guidance to the special panel of masters if, as we expected, the state failed to provide adequate treatment.

Dean and I thought it would be good strategy to show Judge Johnson that the standards for treatment we were urging him to adopt had the support of several broad-based organizations. So we asked him to allow the American Civil Liberties Union, the American Orthopsychiatric Association, and the American Psychological Association to enter the case as friends of the court, and he agreed.

I represented the ACLU. "Ortho" chose as its representative Charles Halpern, a young Washington lawyer who, in the first case of his legal career, had argued the precedent-making case of *Rouse* v. *Cameron*, in which Federal Judge David L. Bazelon first judicially acknowledged that mental patients have a right to adequate treatment. Another Washington lawyer, Jeffrey Bauman, represented the APA. We made Washington our headquarters. Paul Friedman and Ronna Beck, from Halpern's office, rounded out our task force.

Our first step was a two-day tour of Bryce, accompanied by Al Wellner, a psychologist from the APA. George Dean met us at the airport and reported that the previous day two attendants had been caught trying to castrate a seventy-four-year-old patient by pulling on his testicles with a rope (they subsequently received six-month sentences). And a few days earlier Ira Dement, the United States attorney for that area and a friend of Dean's, had cut short his own tour of the hospital when he slipped on a pile of excrement in the middle of a ward corridor.

At Bryce, we split up, each to concentrate on a different ward. I inspected the maximum-security ward and found the patients there so heavily medicated they could barely stand. The ward dayroom had a television set, which an attendant assured me "sometimes" worked. Other than that, there was nothing but a gray metal table and a few empty chairs—no books, magazines, games, or playing cards. The walls were completely bare. None of the patients on the ward were involved in group therapy or individual therapy. About once a month, they were taken outside to a cramped exercise yard. The rest of the time they just sat around, not even talking to each other, waiting to be cured.

Three of the ward's patients had been locked in nine-by-nine-foot solitary isolation cells for eleven days for trying to escape. Each of these cells had a ceiling light bulb, and a mattress and bedding on the floor (no bed frame)—nothing more. The cells, which had no toilets or sinks, gave off an overpowering smell of urine. When my escort, a doctor, turned the keylock and removed two padlocks to let me enter one of the cells, the patient immediately said, "For God's sake, let me out of here! I can't stand this." I entered a second cell, and the patient cried out, "When am I going to get out of here? I feel like an animal in here! This place smells worse than a dog pen."

My escort admitted that the three were locked in isolation not as therapy but as punishment. I asked when they would be released, and he replied that the hospital would "try to review their cases sometime during the next week." But he admitted that they could be held in solitary for weeks, or even months.

Our litigation team compared tour notes and then began interviewing experts, drafting standards, and preparing briefs and reports for the court. At the end of the six-month period, the state submitted a foot-thick report, together with computer print-outs, to support its claim that it had met the court's order to provide adequate treatment. We submitted a counterreport. On December 10, 1971, Judge Johnson ruled that the patients in Bryce were still not receiving adequate treatment, and he ordered both sides to present evidence at trial from which he could determine minimum staff-to-patient ratios and other standards necessary to ensure adequate treatment. For the first time, a federal court would be telling a state, in detail, how to run its mental hospitals.

We knew that Judge Johnson's standards would become the model for right-to-treatment cases throughout the United States. In a sense, our task force was representing not only the patients in Bryce, but also the nearly three-quarters of a million like them in other hospitals across the nation, and the millions that would follow in years to come.

We had less than two months to prepare for trial. Most of that time was consumed in drafting, circulating, and redrafting our proposed standards, and in negotiating with the defendants about which of the standards they would agree not to oppose. By the middle of January, the defendants had stipulated that most of our standards were indeed necessary for adequate treatment. Since the agreed-upon standards would ensure a more active treatment program than existed in most of the nation's mental hospitals, we had already won a great deal. But several of our proposals, including staffing ratios, were still in dispute.

We had hoped to call as witnesses the nation's leading psychiatrists, psychologists, behavioral research analysts, and community facilities experts, but many had prior commitments, so we submitted their depositions instead. This involved considerable travel in the brief time before the hearing. One of the depositions was from Dr. Israel Zwerling, psychiatrist, psychologist, chairman of the department of psychiatry at Einstein College of Medicine, and director of Bronx State Mental Hospital. Bronx State was the only public hospital in the New York City area from which I had not received one patient complaint in three years. Zwerling could be sworn in New York. But Charles Halpern had to fly to Chicago to take the deposition of Dr. Harold M. Visotsky, chairman of the department of psychiatry at Northwestern University Medical School and former director of the Illinois Department of Mental Health. On January 27, just a week before trial, I flew to Burlington, Iowa, to take the deposition of Dr. Walter Fox, past president of the Association of Medical Superintendents of Mental Hospitals and director-elect of the Division of Mental Health Services for the state of Arizona.

The hearing was to begin on February 3, 1972, but our litigation team arrived in Montgomery, Alabama, several days earlier to finish interviewing prospective witnesses and co-ordinate trial strategy. I stayed up until 3:30 A.M. the night before the hearing perfecting an introductory statement. Then Judge Johnson decided he did not need any introductory statements. With his "Are your witnesses ready?" we plunged ahead with the evidence.

George Dean called Dr. Jack Ewalt as the plaintiffs' first witness. Ewalt, chairman of the department of psychiatry at Harvard Medical School, was also a past president of the American Psychiatric Association. Ewalt and our subsequent witnesses supported the depositions of Doctors Visotsky, Zwerling, and Fox, all of whom agreed that the conditions outlined in our standards were necessary for adequate treatment.

The most prominent witness for the defense was Dr. Karl Menninger, who testified that the staffing ratios proposed by the defendants, which were much lower than ours, would nonetheless be adequate. Our experts had proposed a minimum of one psychiatrist for every 30 to 50 patients, but Dr. Menninger testified that one for every 125 patients was enough. Charles Halpern and I were sharing the trial responsibilities, and we had agreed that I would cross-examine Dr. Menninger. But it became clear during his testimony that any attempt to discredit Dr. Menninger, the grand old man of psychiatry, would fail, and might even anger Judge Johnson. Thus, rather than point out, for example, that the director of Bryce State Hospital was Menninger's friend and protégé and a former employee of the Menninger Clinic, I simply told the judge we had no questions. Instead, I waited for Dr. William Tarnower, a psychiatrist on the staff of Menninger's famed clinic, to testify, and then asked him how many psychiatrists the Menninger Clinic employed. The answer —one for every eight patients—made our point, and I sat down.

The case had originally been concerned only with the rights of the mentally ill, but the complaint had recently been amended to include the rights of the mentally retarded. That hearing was set for February 28, and Judge Johnson announced that he would not reach any decision until after the conclusion of this second phase of the case.

Until now, my cases had involved only the mentally ill. I had never even been inside an institution for the retarded. Mental illness and mental retardation are quite different phenomena. The retarded are not mentally ill, but are people whose level of intellectual functioning is lower than average, and who lack the maturity and social skills necessary to adapt to society. If they are severely retarded, they may require intensive training before they can even walk, talk, feed and dress themselves, or go to the toilet. According to George Dean, the 2,400 residents in Partlow State School, Alabama's institution for the retarded, received even less care and treatment than the patients in Bryce. After visiting Partlow, I agreed.

We walked through ward after ward of mentally retarded men, women, and children. Our experts, who toured Partlow with us, told us that with proper education, care, and training, all but a very few of those residents could live in the community. But in Partlow they received no care and no training. There were eighty to ninety of them to a ward, often staffed by only one attendant. Partlow was so crowded that many residents had to sleep on floor mats. The conditions were barbaric. We saw a man who had been locked in solitary confinement for seven years. A little girl in the nonambulatory ward was tied to her bed—otherwise she would try to stand—because there was no one there to catch her if she fell. Agitated residents stuffed dirt and rocks down their throats or lapped garbage water like dogs; we saw one woman in a strait jacket trying to spit the flies out of her mouth. Helpless children lay for hours in pools of urine. Everywhere was hopelessness, neglect, and despair.

At the Partlow hearing the next day, our experts included Gunnar Dybwad, chairman of the sociology department at Brandeis University; Dave Rosen, president-elect of the American Association on Mental Deficiency; Dr. James Clements, vice-president-elect of the AAMD; and Ignacy Goldberg, a professor in the department of special education, Teachers College, Columbia University, and past president of the AAMD.

The United States government, also appearing as a friend of the court, called Dr. Philip Roos, executive director of the National Association for Retarded Children. All these experts supported our proposed standards. The plaintiffs called Linda Glenn, an expert on community facilities, who presented evidence to show that almost all of the Partlow residents could be treated more adequately in the community, and at less cost.

One witness, a University of Alabama student who worked summers at Partlow, testified that attendants had physically beaten and choked patients until they were unconscious, and that such beatings, sometimes with broomsticks, were not uncommon. The acting director of Partlow, an inexperienced but well-intentioned young psychologist, admitted on the witness stand that one resident had died when another resident jammed a water hose up his rectum. Other residents, he conceded, had been scalded to death. And recently a young resident had died of an overdose of medication that he took from an unlocked medicine room. Those deaths, and others, could have been prevented if Partlow had had an adequate staff. The evidence of neglect was so overwhelming that the defendants conceded Partlow was constitutionally inadequate and agreed to virtually all of our newly prepared standards for treatment of the retarded, including the staffing ratios. Judge Johnson gave us two weeks to submit post-trial briefs.

The Partlow hearing disturbed me. If Alabama was representative, institutions for the mentally retarded were worse, if that was possible, than institutions for the mentally ill. There are more than 200,000 mentally retarded persons in public residential institutions, another 60,000 in private facilities, and thousands more on waiting lists.

I flew back to New York and within a week began drafting a complaint challenging the adequacy of treatment at Willowbrook State School for the retarded on Staten Island, the largest such institution in the world.

On April 13, 1972, Judge Johnson reached his decision. In two separate opinions, one for the mentally ill and one for the mentally retarded, he ruled that nearly all of our proposed standards were "both medical and constitutional minimums" which Alabama would have to meet. Those standards, if followed in other states, would cause a revolution in institutional health-care services. Under those standards, for example, Willowbrook would have to employ eighty-seven psychologists; it now has five. In order to meet the standards, states would be forced to discharge vast numbers of inappropriately hospitalized patients. Those who remained would live in a normally furnished homelike environment, retaining all the rights of privacy, communication, and human dignity enjoyed by other citizens. And they would be given individualized programs of treatment, job training, and assistance designed to return them quickly to their communities.

7 / Learn to Labor and to Wait

Let us, then, be up and doing,
With a heart for any fate;
Still achieving, still pursuing,
Learn to labour and to wait.
        —HENRY WADSWORTH LONGFELLOW
        "A Psalm of Life"

Edna Dalton Long, mental patient, was paid nothing for the six-teen years she labored against her will in the kitchens and corri-dors of Harlem Valley State Hospital. Patient labor—on the farm, in the laundry, on the grounds, and in the boiler room—ran the hospital. There were rewards for the "good worker": transfer to a better ward, permission to roam the grounds, an oc-casional weekend pass, and, always, promises that a co-operative attitude would bring him one step closer to discharge. For Edna, that long-awaited day came in April of 1967, when she was in her late sixties, too old at last to work.

Edna was born in 1901 of a Scottish father and a French mother. She graduated from high school and worked as a bookkeeper in Lowell, Massachusetts. At night, she improved her business skills at an extension course in accounting offered by Boston University. She then moved to California and finished one year of college at UCLA. In 1938, she moved to New York City and shortly thereafter married Fred Long, a railroad worker. It was then that her troubles began. Seven times in ten years she was found intoxicated in public places—in theaters, subways, on the streets—and was taken by the police to either Bellevue, Central Islip, Pilgrim, or Kings Park Hospital, where she stayed until she was sober and promised abstinence. The diagnosis was always the same: "Psychosis due to alcohol."

May 2, 1951, was the date of her first admission to Harlem Valley. On December 9, 1951, she left the hospital on "convalescent care status," but three days later she "got drunk and intoxicated, fell on the street," and was returned. Discharged in July of 1952, she was back again in August and was assigned to Building 28, her home for the next sixteen years.

The diagnosis, again, was "Psychosis due to alcohol," but the hospital records reveal that throughout her hospitalization there was "no clear evidence of a psychosis." Her I.Q. of 134 was "superior," and she did "not appear to be irrational or detached from reality." To the contrary, as Dr. A. F. Rizzolo noted in her record only two days after her admission:

RETENTION AND IMMEDIATE RECALL: Excellent; able to do ten digits forward and eight in reversed order.

COUNTING AND CALCULATION: Excellent.

MENTAL GRASP AND CAPACITY: Well-retained.

ORIENTATION: Excellent for time, place, and person.

RECENT MEMORY: Excellent.

REMOTE MEMORY: Apparently intact.

And the hospital found that Edna Dalton Long was "not dangerous to herself or others."

It is difficult to understand why she was kept so long. Perhaps the hospital, convinced she would return again—and soon—thought it senseless to discharge her, at least until she had gained enough "insight" to stop "minimizing her past difficulties" with alcohol. Instead, she continued "to rationalize her behavior, to deny her illness and need for hospitalization," and remained "hostile, suspicious, and persistent in demanding her release." To the hospital, her insistence that she was "imprisoned" for no good reason indicated she was "paranoid toward hospital authorities." To her, the evidence of imprisonment was clear enough: she rarely talked with a psychiatrist and received no psychotherapy, either group or individual; except once during the first year, her alcoholism problem was not even discussed. She objected most of all to her "work assignments," which she considered "demeaning and beneath my abilities."

Upon admission, Nurse O'Brien had asked whether Edna Long was a paying or a nonpaying patient, explaining that the latter were "expected" to work. The following day, Edna was roused at 5:30 A.M. by the morning attendant, who instructed her to care for the elderly and incontinent female patients, demonstrating how to lift them from their beds, wash them with a sponge, remove the urine-soaked sheets, change their clothes and linen, feed them, and wheel them to the dayroom. For two months she tended her listless charges until, unable to endure the fecal smells and other details of the job, she begged to be relieved. The hospital relented and another patient took her place.

Edna Long's next assignment was working behind the steam table in the employees' dining room three meals a day, seven days a week, loading and unloading dishes, scouring vats, and polishing the brass-capped table legs between meals. She complained and was shifted to the clothes room in Building 25, where, for eight hours a day, she folded, sorted, and dispatched clean clothes. Soon she was back at the steam table, this time for two meals a day, six days a week, and she worked there for the next ten years. In her spare time, she continued to be "helpful on the ward with elderly ladies" and with the "helpless patients, seeing that they are clean by changing their clothing and combing their hair."

Exhausted by her labors, and furious that she had to work for her "jailer," Edna Long told the staff that she would not work any longer. A few days later her husband came to visit and showed her a letter from a Harlem Valley doctor which rejected his request that Edna be discharged, pointing out that she had been "unco-operative" toward her work assignments. Twice Edna attempted to interest the courts in her release, with no success. Convinced she would never be free until she pleased her "captors," she returned to the kitchen.

There were other periods of rebellion. Seven times in three years she refused to work. But the attendants, whose work load was increased by her recalcitrance, threatened to enter unfavorable notations in her record, took away her cigarettes, ignored her physical complaints (she frequently suffered headaches and pains in her lower back and legs), turned off the ward TV in the middle of whatever program she happened to be watching, and in general made life on the ward so disagreeable that she was eventually forced to choose the drudgery of the kitchen over the antagonism of the ward.

In June of 1964, Edna Long began "working in the sewing room in the a.m. daily." In October, she "complained of not being able to see out of her right eye," but continued to work mornings in the sewing room, visiting the eye clinic in the afternoon. Her supervising psychiatrist, Dr. Anna Bauman, told her she had a cataract, but it was not until April of 1965, six months after she had complained, that her assignment to the sewing room was terminated.

For the remainder of 1965, she worked evenings in the diet

kitchen and, during the day, using an electric floor polisher, handled "the polishing on the ward" while "hoping to get her sight back in her right eye." Following a glaucoma operation and a one-month recuperation, she was back at work waxing and polishing the ward floors by day and "cleaning the offices in the Administration Building in the evening."

On April 18, 1967, the staff said good-by to Edna Dalton Long and put her on a bus to New York City. The reason for her discharge, refused so many times before, is unclear. The hospital record does not indicate any change in her mental condition. Her guess is that she was getting too old (sixty-six) to be an effective laborer, and that her continuing eye problems (she had two more operations after she was released) made her more of a bother than she was worth. Less than a week after discharge, she found modest employment as a bookkeeper, which kept her going for two years, until her eyes and health gave out. That was when she came to me.

Edna Dalton Long was short, almost plump, with a cheerful face and a light, responsive manner. She had bright red lipstick and rouged cheeks, and was wearing costume jewelry and a short blond wig. At first, however, I noticed only her eyes— enormously magnified and elongated behind thick bifocal lenses, and tired.

Too proud for welfare, too old to work; what was she to do? I asked if she had any savings. With surprising bitterness she snapped, "No. They took everything I had, every penny."

Before commitment to Harlem Valley, Edna Long had set aside a few thousand dollars for her retirement. During the first eleven years of hospitalization, she had prudently managed her own business affairs by correspondence and had watched her savings grow to almost $9,000.

In June of 1960, her husband died, leaving her a small pension from the Railroad Retirement Board. (The hospital did not notify Edna of his death for three weeks. She then learned, to her

dismay, that the state had buried him in a pauper's grave in pot-
ter's field and kept his lump-sum burial benefit.) Two years later,
the hospital decided that it wanted her money. On June 1, 1962,
Dr. Lawrence P. Roberts, the director of Harlem Valley, petitioned a court to declare Edna Dalton Long incompetent and to
appoint a committee to manage her property "for the purpose of
having said property, so far as the same shall be required for that
purpose, applied for the maintenance and support of said alleged
incompetent in a state institution." In other words, the state
wanted to take her savings as reimbursement for the costs of her
involuntary hospitalization.

The state could simply have sued for the money, but that
would have taken time and, conceivably, the state might have
lost. Indeed, I believe the state would have lost. After all, Edna
did not receive any treatment, and the forced labor she performed
for the hospital was probably worth more than the cost of her
food, clothing, and shelter. It was easier and less risky, from the
state's point of view, to entrust her money to a committee, which
would in turn give it to the state. But before a committee could
legally take control of Edna Long's money, she would have to be
found incompetent to manage her property. Of course, she had
already been found to be mentally ill, but a person can be mentally ill without being mentally incompetent. However, it is clear
from Edna Long's hospital record and from the sequence of
events leading to the appointment of her committee that no one
really cared whether she was incompetent or not.

On April 11, 1962, H. Elman, a reimbursement agent in the
Department of Mental Hygiene's New York City office, sent a
form letter to Dr. Roberts, which read: "The financial status of
the above patient is such that committee proceedings are felt to
be necessary. Please complete this form and return it to me so
that the Attorney General will be in a position to institute such
proceedings." The form did not even ask whether Roberts
thought Edna Long was competent or incompetent.

On May 3, 1962, after receiving the information, Elman forwarded it to the attorney general "in order that you may proceed to have a committee appointed for the above-named patient." The attorney general then drafted a petition which he forwarded to Dr. Roberts, the hospital director, for his signature. The petition contained the allegation, required by statute, that Edna Dalton Long was incompetent, but the allegation was so obviously taken from a form book that it described Edna Long as "incompetent to manage *himself*," or "*his*" property. Roberts later admitted under oath that if he had "noticed" the "himself" language on the printed form, he would have corrected it. But he did not. Instead, he promptly signed and returned the petition without adding or changing anything, and the attorney general filed it with the court.

Later, Roberts admitted under oath that he had "found" Edna Long to be incompetent without even a personal examination. He did not remember ever discussing Edna's competence, or lack of it, with any other doctor. He claimed to have reached his conclusion after spending a half hour or so looking through her hospital record. Much of her record consisted of "ward matter of nonmedical personnel," all of which, said Roberts, was "taken into consideration." In other words, the evidence of incompetence came from the random notes of untrained and poorly educated laymen, none of whom had been asked to evaluate Edna Long's competence. Roberts simply ignored the countervailing evidence of her superior I.Q., her year of college, her business background as a bookkeeper, and her successful management of her affairs. Roberts admitted that he had "nothing to do with preparing the petition," and that the allegation of incompetence was prepared by the attorney general's office, without consultation with the hospital staff. That was the way it was "always" done. The inference was clear: Edna Long had been labeled incompetent so that the state could get her money. So had thousands like her. That they were not really incompetent was a mere detail.

By July 24, it was all over. Judge Bernard Newman read the

petition and decided it was unnecessary to bring Edna Long before him to hear what she might have to say. Relying on the allegation of incompetence that the attorney general had so scrupulously provided, Judge Newman found her incompetent and appointed Demarest J. Hahn, a lawyer, to be her committee (in such cases, a "committee" can be only one person), authorizing him to reimburse the state for the costs of her hospitalization.

Hahn did a poor job of managing Edna Long's estate. Because he transferred her assets from a savings account to a checking account, she lost almost $2,000 in interest. Because he failed for two years to file the annual report required by statute of all committees, the Railroad Retirement Board stopped sending her husband's monthly pension payments. Eventually the situation became so intolerable that even the attorney general "recommended surcharges against the committee." The court, however, permitted Hahn to resign, and to keep the $730 he had deducted from Edna's estate as the commission and fees for his services.

On April 10, 1967, the court appointed Edward Pious, another lawyer, as the successor committee, though there was, in fact, no need for a successor committee. On March 1, 1967, Dr. Harry Bittle had told Edna Long she would be discharged as soon as living arrangements could be made. Notification of her impending discharge was sent to the attorney general, together with the hospital's opinion that she was now considered "competent to manage her own affairs." The attorney general, however, did not relay that information to the court. Edna Long could have told the court that she was about to be discharged, except that she knew nothing about the proceeding to discharge Hahn and appoint Pious until it was over. And so, on April 18, 1967, one week after Pious assumed control of her estate, Edna Long was discharged.

After checking into the Isaac Hooper Home on Manhattan's Second Avenue, she went immediately to Pious, asking that he return all the "financial assets, taken from me while I was imprisoned, together with accruals and all other monies collected in my name—and every penny of interest on all." Pious refused to turn over what was left of her estate unless she signed a formal release discharging any claims she might have against Hahn and himself. Angered, she left, and he continued to control her assets, collecting commissions for his efforts, for three more years.

Edna Long did not know it, but I had been waiting for a case like hers. I had read—in *The Trouble with Lawyers*, by Murray Teigh Bloom—a castigation of the committee system in New York, which pointed out that it was not uncommon for mental patients to lose 80 per cent of their assets at the hands of committees ostensibly appointed for their protection (Edna Long had lost $8,000, almost 86 per cent of her estate). Pious was named in Bloom's book as one of the most frequently appointed lawyers in New York incompetency proceedings. And I had recently talked with Dr. F. Lewis Bartlett, a Pennsylvania psychiatrist who had started a one-man crusade to abolish what he called "institutional peonage," or forced labor, in mental hospitals. Edna Long's case raised both issues.

For jurisdictional reasons, I decided to file two lawsuits—one in the state court of claims requesting compensation for the labor Edna Long had performed at Harlem Valley, and another in federal court challenging the committee system.

The state case was filed in December, 1969, and took fifteen months to work its way up the court of claims' trial calendar. Then, in March of 1971, less than two weeks before we were scheduled to begin trial, the state made a belated motion to dismiss Edna Long's forced-labor claim on the ground that the work assignments were part of her "therapy," and thus, even if excessive, were matters of "professional medical judgment," for which, even if erroneous, the state was not responsible. The sole support for that position was a three-page affidavit from Dr. Anna Bauman, a psychiatrist at Harlem Valley, who had been in charge of Building 28, where Edna Long lived, from November, 1963, until Edna's discharge three and a half years later. Dr. Bauman claimed that no work was assigned in Building 28 without her approval.

William Pratt, an attorney in private practice who volunteered his services in this case (and in the Summers case described in the next chapter) helped me put together a sixty-one-page brief in opposition to the state's motion to dismiss. We first pointed out that the "professional judgment" defense, even if valid, covered only the last few years of Edna Long's hospitalization. No doctor claimed to have exercised professional judgment over her work assignments from 1951 to 1963. More important, on the basis of affidavits from our own experts, we challenged the state's assertion that the work Edna Long had done was therapeutic; it was the opinion of our psychiatrists that the work was antitherapeutic.

Dr. F. Lewis Bartlett is the country's leading psychiatric expert on "institutional peonage," or, in legal terms, involuntary servitude. In November of 1969, the United States Senate recognized his expertise by asking him to testify before the Senate Subcommittee on the Constitutional Rights of the Mentally Ill. After reviewing Edna Long's hospital records, Bartlett concluded that the work she had performed was cost saving and performed for the hospital's benefit, not hers. She had proved such a valuable worker that even though her mental condition was stable, she had been kept for sixteen years. That is, she had become as indispensable as the attendant on her ward, or the ward nurse, and the hospital gave no more thought to her discharge than to theirs.

Dr. Walter Fox, a psychiatrist who in 1969–70 was the president of the Association of Medical Superintendents of Mental Hospitals, examined her records and concluded that the work she had performed was "not therapy," but "exploitation. . . . In other words, she worked there, not for her own well-being, but for that of the hospital." Dr. James Finkelstein (like Fox, a diplomate in psychiatry of the American Board of Psychiatry and

Neurology) asserted that Edna Long's work assignments "could not have any therapeutic value." And Bart K. Lubow, a research scientist who had achieved national recognition for his empirical research on patient work programs, stated that "the work she performed while a patient at Harlem Valley Hospital could in no way be considered therapeutic and very likely may have had an antitherapeutic effect which contributed to her extended period of hospitalization." Clearly, we had the experts on our side.

The state's motion was argued in Poughkeepsie, New York, on April 20, 1971, before Judge Milton Alpert. The issues were important. If we prevailed, it would be the first time in United States history that a mental patient would recover damages for involuntary labor. Such a victory could shake the structure of the mental hospital system, which required patient labor for its existence. On May 7, Judge Alpert ruled in our favor on the legal issues and set the case down for a trial. Our claim did, in fact, state a "cause of action." If we could prove at trial the facts we had alleged in our claim, we would win. The state immediately filed a notice of appeal, but five months later, on October 14, 1971, it withdrew the appeal and announced it was ready for trial. Apparently the state had decided that Judge Alpert's decision was correct on the law; to win at all, the state would have to win on the facts.

The facts, however, were on our side. After the state withdrew its appeal, Bill Pratt and I took the deposition of Dr. Anna Bauman, the Harlem Valley psychiatrist who had submitted the affidavit claiming that Edna Long's work assignments were part of a therapeutic program. Testifying reluctantly, Dr. Bauman conceded the truth of most of our factual allegations.

There had been only two psychiatrists, Dr. Bauman and her assistant, to treat the 650 patients in Building 28. Dr. Bauman had spent most of her time answering mail and attending to administrative matters. Once or twice a week she made rounds, which gave her an hour or two to inspect the patients as she went from ward to ward. By her estimate—which I thought was high—

she spent one-third of her time, and the other psychiatrist one-half of his time, in direct patient contact. In effect, the state provided less than one full-time psychiatrist to treat the 650 patients in Building 28—or, to put it another way, one psychiatrist for every 800 patients.

Dr. Bauman and her assistant left the building at night, on weekends, and for vacations, as did the building's only nurse. There were only thirty-six attendants, twelve for each shift, or one attendant for every fifty-five patients. It was easy to see why the hospital needed patient labor.

Dr. Bauman conceded that Edna Long had received no group or individual psychotherapy. Her therapy had consisted solely of medication and work.

Dr. Bauman said that if patients "didn't work they didn't get open ward cards or ground privileges." Working patients could "go for walks" or "to activities," and could "have more freedom." They were also transferred to "more pleasant wards." Frequently, Edna Long had "refused to work," thus losing her privileges until she changed her mind.

The psychiatrist also testified that Edna Long was not physically dangerous to herself or others, that her mental problem was only a "moderate case" of brain deterioration due to excessive drinking, that "she still had her intellectual faculties," that she "didn't show the signs of permanent deterioration," that "she was in contact with reality," and that "she had a superior intelligence." The conclusion seemed inescapable: Edna Long was kept for sixteen years because she was a good worker.

She had worked mainly in the employees' dining room, but Dr. Bauman "didn't actually assign her there." When Dr. Bauman came to Building 28, Edna had been working in the dining room for many years, and Dr. Bauman "just allowed her to continue there." The hospital record did not show who made the initial assignment to the dining room; it might have been an attendant.

In order to invoke the "professional judgment" defense, the

state had claimed that every work assignment at Harlem Valley was approved by a doctor. But Dr. Bauman's testimony didn't quite say that: "As a matter of fact, when a doctor makes an assignment he only assigns the *area* of the assignment. Like the dining room." The "type of work" the patient would perform in that area was "left up to" the nonprofessional staff. Dr. Bauman "didn't evaluate the type of work" Edna Long performed in the dining room, even though the doctor knew some of the jobs in the dining room "might have been better for her than others."

The professional judgment defense also seemed inapplicable to Edna Long's work in the sewing room, because Dr. Bauman admitted it would have been "a better practice to terminate her assignment in the sewing room as soon as [I] learned she was having eye problems."

Since Dr. Bauman was the only professional who claimed any knowledge of Edna Long's work assignments, it seemed to me that the professional judgment defense would not stand up in court. Encouraged by the weakness of the state's defense, we were eager to go to trial. Unfortunately, because of the state's appeal we lost our place on the trial calendar and had to wait several more months for the trial.

Our expert witnesses included Doctors Fox and Bartlett, Dr. Ian Alger, representing the American Orthopsychiatric Association, Allen Williams, executive director of the New York State Psychological Association, and Irving Chase, president of the National Association for Mental Health, all of whom testified that Edna's work had been good for the state, but not for her. Judge Daniel Becker reserved decision, giving the state one month to round up witnesses for its side. After the decision will come the inevitable appeals, to the appellate division and the Court of Appeals, and then, perhaps, to the United States Supreme Court. Thus, at this writing, I cannot tell you whether Edna Dalton Long will win or lose.

I can tell you that hospital administrators are worried. Cases like this are beginning to spring up elsewhere. And the federal government is beginning to insist that, in at least some circumstances, patients be paid for the labor they perform. Maybe Edna Long will be the first to win. Maybe not. But someone will win, and hospital slavery will end.

So much for Edna's state case, challenging involuntary servitude. Her federal suit, challenging the committee system, was filed on August 8, 1969.

New York law recognizes a substantial difference between mental incompetence and mental illness. A mentally healthy person may, because of old age or physical handicap, be incompetent to look after his business affairs. Conversely, a mentally ill person who requires hospitalization may be fully competent to manage his business affairs. Fewer than 10 per cent of the mental patients in New York's state hospitals have been found incompetent. Nevertheless, the procedure for determining the business competence of a mental patient is very different from that for determining the business competence of a nonpatient.

The procedure for nonpatients requires a verified, or sworn, petition that alleges incompetence and also includes sufficient facts to support the allegation. Proceedings against a patient can be instituted by an unsworn petition containing only allegations, with no facts to support them. More important, the nonpatient has an absolute right to a jury trial and cannot be found incompetent unless twelve jurors agree. The patient has no right to a jury trial, or even to a hearing before a judge. The judge can simply read the unsworn petition, accept the allegations as true, and find the patient incompetent, without giving him an opportunity to prove his competence—without even giving him notice that his competence is in question. That is what has happened to thousands of patients, including Edna Dalton Long, who first learned of the incompetency proceeding three months after it was over, when she wrote to a Boston attorney asking him to collect and bank the proceeds of a matured life insurance policy, only to discover that the proceeds had already been paid to "her committee."

Jonathan Weiss and Mark Wurm, two lawyers from the Columbia Center on Social Welfare Policy and Law, a law reform project funded by the Office of Economic Opportunity, volunteered to help challenge the committee system and together we sketched out our three main arguments.

First, we said, everyone, even a mental patient, is entitled to his day in court. Since Edna Long had not been given notice or an opportunity to be heard, the proceeding violated her Fourteenth Amendment right to "due process."

Second, it was a violation of Edna's Fourteenth Amendment right to the "equal protection of the law" to deprive her, a patient, of procedural protections—for example, the right to jury trial—that were available to nonpatients, especially since the issue—is the person incompetent?—was exactly the same, whether the person was a mental patient or not.

Our final argument was that no matter how fair the procedures, it was unconstitutional to label a person incompetent and take away his assets when the purpose of the proceeding was not to preserve those assets until the person had regained competence, but to spend them. In a subsequent deposition, Dr. Roberts, the director of Harlem Valley, admitted that he did not know of a single instance in which Edna Long had squandered or mismanaged her assets, and that he had not bothered to ask his staff if they knew how well she managed her business affairs. He did not even know, when he signed the petition, that she had a bank account.

When Roberts was asked to locate in the hospital record a single incident suggesting to him that Edna was incompetent, he referred to the notes he had assembled in preparation for the deposition, and chose the following:

A note of December the 13th, 1960, from Dr. Podnieks, by Dr. Podnieks, the hospital received from the Railroad Retirement Board application forms for eventual benefits where the patient has to give some data about her life and previous work.

When interviewed for this reason, the patient states she would not give any data to the physician to be entered in the forms because she wants her lawyer to do so.

It seemed to me quite sensible of Edna Long to prefer the advice of a lawyer over that of a physician before she filled out the legal forms submitted to her by the Railroad Retirement Board. Aware that his example was not persuasive, Dr. Roberts immediately turned to the most bizarre incident he could find, one that "undoubtedly had a part in my decision that she was incompetent":

The patient was having a disturbed episode. She was sitting on the floor, dazed, talking to herself and staring into space. Then sitting on the toilet with her back between her legs, with paper and dollar bills in the water. Transferred to a closed ward.

It seemed to me more likely that whoever wrote that note was incompetent—it was difficult to imagine what the writer had in mind when he described Edna as sitting on the toilet "with her back between her legs." The sloppiness of that observation cast doubt on the accuracy of the entire note. But even if the incident had occurred, it did not prove that Edna Long was incompetent. First, there was no indication *why* she was "disturbed"— perhaps an attendant or another patient had hit her. Perhaps she had fallen, or been given too much medication. Second, there was no indication that the "paper and dollar bills" belonged to her. Third, the note described an isolated incident that had occurred fifteen months before Roberts signed the petition alleging she was incompetent.

Furthermore, when pressed, Roberts conceded that he did not remember having read those notes before he signed the petition.

In fact, he was not certain that he had ever read through Edna Long's hospital record.

We asked the federal court to set aside the adjudication of incompetence and order the defendants (Hahn, Pious,* Roberts, and Alan D. Miller, the Commissioner of Mental Hygiene) to return all the money they had expended from Edna Long's estate, including the committee expenses (commissions, fees, bond premiums, and the like), none of which would have been incurred had she been permitted to manage her own affairs.

The defendants made a motion to dismiss the complaint, contending that the federal court lacked jurisdiction and that, in any event, Edna Long *had* been given notice of the incompetency proceeding, and by failing to request a personal appearance before the judge had waived any objections she might have had. Instead of holding a hearing to determine whether Edna Long had or had not received notice, Judge Irving Ben Cooper accepted the state's version of the facts and dismissed the complaint. He went further: he ruled that the complaint did not raise "substantial" constitutional questions and that the federal court lacked jurisdiction.

We appealed Judge Cooper's decision to the United States Court of Appeals for the Second Circuit. The appeal took a year, but in February of 1971, the appellate court granted it by reversing Judge Cooper and remanding the case for trial on the merits. The three appellate judges agreed that the constitutional questions were substantial, and that it had been improper for Judge Cooper to accept the state's version of the disputed facts without giving us an opportunity to disprove them. More important, they agreed that even if Edna Long had received notice, this would not "automatically resolve the constitutional issue. Because of a mental hospital inmate's alleged condition, it may well be that

---

* Pious was subsequently dropped as a defendant when he agreed to file a state court accounting.

personal notice to the inmate is insufficient and that independent guardians *ad litem* [for that case] should be appointed in all cases for such inmates."

The appellate court was suggesting that every incompetency proceeding might require the mandatory appointment of a guardian or lawyer to represent the alleged incompetent, and might also require a mandatory court hearing. Such requirements would make the incompetency procedure much less convenient for the state. And if doctors actually had to appear in court to justify their allegations of incompetence, the number of frivolous incompetency proceedings would decline markedly.

The state was so annoyed by the appellate court's decision that it took the unusual step of filing a petition for rehearing, asking the appellate court to reverse its own decision. The appellate court responded by not only affirming the first decision, but also issuing a supplemental decision that afforded alleged incompetents even more protection than the first decision had provided.

Although we had won an important round, we still had to go back before Judge Cooper and persuade him that our arguments were not only substantial but compelling. Cooper would be antagonistic toward us—our appellate brief had treated his decision roughly. On the other hand, it was evident from the tone of the appellate decision that the higher court was extremely sympathetic to our arguments. Fearing a second reversal, Cooper might now be more sympathetic to our complaint.

Months would go by before the trial was completed, but the Department of Mental Hygiene, sensing ultimate defeat, caved in and proposed a new statute that would give allegedly incompetent patients most of the procedural protections we were demanding. The new statute would help others, but it would not help Edna Long, and she needed help badly.

Because she refused to accept welfare and was too old to work, she could afford nothing better than a decrepit one-room flat in a run-down section of Coney Island. The tiny room held a shabby bed, a sink, a refrigerator, a small coffee table, and a makeshift closet consisting of a curtain hung diagonally across one corner. The room was hot and dark (the only window opened on a ventilation shaft, with no light or view), and so cramped that by stretching my arms I could almost reach from wall to wall.

One day, while preparing for the trial, I decided to pay Edna Long a surprise visit. She apologized for the clutter as she let me in. I noticed an old woman in a black shawl sitting quietly in the corner sipping tea. That was Edna's "friend," she told me. The old woman spoke only French, and Edna spoke only English, but twice a week they visited each other, occasionally attempting a rough communication with gestures and exclamations. For the most part, though, they sat together wordlessly sharing the hardness of their lives.

8 / Psychiatrists
Don't Believe in Prayer

Mary Summers was an urban hermit. Beginning in 1966, she rarely left her room in New York's Hotel Pierrepont. Except for a daily hot meal ordered from the hotel coffee shop, she lived on canned food, Arnold's bread, jams, and preserves. She had few acquaintances and fewer friends. Perhaps her life was not particularly full or happy—she herself called it "odd" and "restricted"— but it was *her* life, and she had a plan to make it better.

In 1958, when she was forty-eight, having decided to face up to her "problem," as she called it, Miss Summers became a devoted follower of Christian Science. As her faith developed, she read deeply in Christian Science literature and began to entertain practitioners weekly in her hotel room; some of them became good friends. She read the Bible daily, and for the first time in many years she began to venture out more frequently, sometimes by day and for longer periods at a time. She even met a man. Theirs was a brief and modest romance, but it was more than she had known before.

The improvement in her social relations eventually encouraged Mary Summers to tackle her "other problem," a serious diuretic condition that obliged her to make frequent trips down the dingy hotel corridor to the bathroom shared by everyone on her floor. To her neighbors, it seemed that she was always there. At first they had only muttered among themselves, but later they began to hide the toilet paper, turn over the waste basket, or leave behind an unflushed toilet when they heard her coming. A few even screamed at her in the hall and pounded on her door. In response she turned up her radio—partly to drown them out and partly to retaliate for their abuse.

Something had to be done. On the advice of her Christian Science practitioner, she called the Department of Social Services and requested a room with a private bath. She was on welfare, and had been for almost twelve years, ever since her small inheritance ran out. Miss Summers told Mrs. Brown, her caseworker, that she was diuretic and that the bickering on her floor could be avoided only if she had her own bathroom. Mrs. Brown said the Welfare Department would look into it, but months went by and nothing happened. When Mary Summers called again, she was told that a private bath required a special allotment, which could be granted only on the recommendation of a doctor or a psychiatrist. Followers of Christian Science are less opposed to verbal or psychiatric examinations than to physical examinations, so Miss Summers asked to see a welfare psychiatrist.

In late 1966, Mrs. Brown came to her room with a psychiatrist, Dr. Robert Reich, who conducted a brief interview. Another year of bickering and recriminations went by at the Hotel Pierrepont as Miss Summers's request for a private bath—assisted perhaps by her complaints to the mayor—worked its way up through successive layers of approval in the welfare hierarchy.

Finally, on April 1, 1968, Mr. Karen, her new caseworker, arrived in a taxi and took Mary Summers and her few possessions to the King Edward Hotel, near Times Square in Manhattan. The small, shabby room she was shown, though it had a private bath, was located in the rear of the hotel, directly facing an adjoining building. There was no view and little light. Miss Summers protested. Mr. Karen asked the hotel clerk if any other rooms were available, and the clerk showed them one with a private bath in the front of the hotel. The rent was slightly higher, but Mr. Karen agreed that it was within the budgetary allotment, and the rent was paid for the month of April.

When, on May 2, Mary Summers attempted to pay her rent for the coming month, she was told by the assistant hotel manager that she would have to move to a less desirable room—front rooms, she now learned, were for transients, not "permanents." After making a brief telephone call to Mr. Karen for help—he told her to "do anything the hotel wants you to do"—Miss Summers said she would not move and locked herself in her room.

Two hours later, several police officers and two hospital attendants broke through the door. The attendants laced her in a strait jacket and carried her to an ambulance. Accompanied by two police officers, she was taken to the psychiatric ward of Bellevue Hospital, where she was admitted as an emergency patient. One of the officers turned over to Bellevue a letter from the Welfare Department written by Dr. Reich six weeks earlier, while Mary Summers was still living at the Hotel Pierrepont.

Admitting Psychiatrist
Kings County Hospital

March 21, 1968

Miss Mary Summers, of 55 Pierrepont Street, is a 58 year old woman, who is continuing to be disruptive in her hotel. She plays the radio all night and guards the public bathroom claiming it is her own. She has not washed in five years and her appearance is totally dirty and disheveled. She has been unable to leave her room for some years and the hotel has been sending food to her room. She has refused medical help of any kind. She has been sending letters to the Mayor's Committee demanding a room with a bath, but despite attempts by the department to help her move, she has been unable to leave the hotel room or to clean herself up so that she could be acceptable in a public hotel. There are no relatives who can help her and we feel that in her present condition she is a danger to herself in that if no food is brought to her she will starve, as well as her argumentative behavior, and the guarding of the bathroom make it utterly impossible to live with others.

I would, therefore, recommend that she be sent to Kings County Hospital for evaluation and treatment for this chronic problem which has grown worse over the years.

A Bellevue employee waved the Reich letter in Miss Summers's face, but would not let her read it. The Reich letter is typical of many written by institutional psychiatrists in that it has a social goal in mind—in this case, the removal of Miss Summers from society. Because such reports are goal oriented, they invent and exaggerate—Miss Summers admitted to me that she was unkempt, but denied the claim that she had not washed in five years. Moreover, such letters omit entirely any detail that might defeat the goal. Why not mention the antagonism of the other residents, for example, or that Miss Summers had a legitimate reason for her frequent trips to the bathroom, or that she had refused medical help because of her religious beliefs? Dr. Reich's suggestion that Mary Summers might be a danger to herself was gratuitous—the New York statute under which she was hospitalized authorized the involuntary hospitalization of the most harmless of persons. Worse, the letter was deliberately misleading. Anyone who read it would suppose she was close to starvation and survived only because of occasional food baskets pressed on her by a humanitarian hotel management. Dr. Reich knew she was five feet, three inches tall and weighed 190 pounds —hardly the statistics of starvation—and he knew the hotel sent food to her room only because she ordered and paid for it. These facts, however, were not mentioned.

The date of the letter was March 21, 1968, six weeks before the emergency admission to Bellevue. A lot can happen in six weeks. If anyone had bothered to ask, Miss Summers could have said that between then and the date of her admission she had moved to the King Edward Hotel, where she had a room with a private bath (thus no longer "guarding the public bathroom") and was getting along well with the other residents. But no one bothered to ask, neither the Bellevue social worker in the admissions office who jotted down her name, age, address, and religion, nor the doctor she saw for less than a minute (he asked to take her blood pressure, she refused, he left). An attendant took her to a ward, a full-fledged patient now, though she still had not been given a psychiatric examination.

From her account, it is not difficult to visualize what happened next. A nurse approaches the gray bench on which she is sitting. "Come on now, Miss Summers. It's time to take your pill."

"I don't want any pill. It's against my religious beliefs. I don't even want to be here. I am being held here against my will."

"Just take your pill. It will make you well so that you can go home."

"I'm not sick. I don't need any pill. And even if I were sick I wouldn't take that pill. I believe in healing by prayer."

"Look, it's the doctor's orders. Everybody has to take their pill. It's not going to hurt you. It's good for you. It's just a tranquilizer. It will calm you down and help you get to sleep."

"I don't want to go to sleep. I just want to get out of here."

"Well, if you won't take it orally, we'll have to give you an injection."

"You can't do that to me. I'm a Christian Scientist."

"Are you going to take your pill or not?"

"No, I will not."

And so she got the shot intramuscularly, meaning that the needle was injected not just under the skin, but deep into the muscle. On May 3, 4, and 5, more medication was given, sometimes by injection, sometimes under threat of injection. Then came May 6. Mary Summers had been at Bellevue five days. The mental hygiene law requires that patients be notified of their legal rights within five days after admission—no point in "stirring them up" sooner, a psychiatrist once told me. Miss Summers's hospital record contained a "Notice of Rights" dated May 6, five days after her admission, but she denies ever having seen it. The notice stated that two doctors had examined her and certified that she was mentally ill. It stated also that an application for her admission to a state mental hospital (Bellevue is a city hospital) had been signed, and that she would be transferred to Central Islip State Hospital on May 10, 1968. In fact, Miss Summers had not been examined by one doctor, much less two. The next day, May 7, she was examined by Doctors Grant and Ollins, who, as predicted in the notice of rights, found her mentally ill and signed a certificate, dated May 7, to that effect. And on May 10, an application for her admission to Central Islip was, in fact, signed by an assistant hospital administrator.

How did the hospital administration know on May 6, the date of the notice, that two doctors would later find Mary Summers mentally ill, that on May 10 an application for her admission would be signed, and that an order authorizing her transfer to Central Islip would be executed, as it was, on May 9? The answer is simple. Mary Summers had been brought to Bellevue by the police accompanied by a complaint from the Welfare Department. Bellevue could no more discharge her to the custody of the Welfare Department than it could return a runaway teen-ager to the parents who brought him to the hospital. Of course, the hospital administration could not have known on May 6 that Mary Summers had a mental problem, but it certainly knew she was a social problem. In the receiving wards of a busy city hospital, the distinction is easily obscured. The examination was meant to confirm what the administration already knew: that this social problem, because of the agencies involved, could not quickly be resolved. Thus Mary Summers became a sacrifice to bureaucratic expediency.

Nor did she cease to be a social problem after her arrival at Central Islip. There, too, according to the hospital records, she showed her indignation,

due to the fact that she is a Christian Scientist and is being forced to take medication. She is constantly berating the hospital and officials for violating her personal rights and privileges as a human being and as a Christian Scientist. She says she will seek court action to get her out and that she would fight these violations, to try to attain a victory on behalf of human rights for an American citizen and specifically for the beliefs of all Christian Scientists.

Like every other new patient, soon after she arrived she was taken to a room, placed in a chair, and told to smile for the camera. She refused, and also objected to being fingerprinted, protesting that she was no "common criminal." She was sent back to her ward and given an injection, accompanied by a threat of additional injections if she continued to be "stubborn." Then she was returned to the photography room, where an attendant took her unsmiling photograph and pushed her hand into the ink smear, rolling her fingers over the print blotter. She was then sent back to her ward and her prints forwarded to the New York State Identification and Intelligence System. NYSIIS is the state agency that stores the fingerprints of all criminals—and mental patients—and sends them on to law enforcement agencies, the Hack License Bureau (see the next chapter), and other public employers. That was that.

Not much happened for the next month or so, except that the tranquilizers forced upon her caused a drug reaction in Mary Summers that lowered her blood pressure to a potentially dangerous 90/60. Nurses were told to "monitor her pressure three times a day" and to "refer to M.D." if she got any worse. Nothing else broke the daily routine.

Halfway through June, a doctor asked her to agree to remain in the hospital as a voluntary patient. She refused. Miss Summers was told that if she did not sign in as a voluntary, the court would commit her for another six months; if she signed, she would be released in a month. She signed. Because she was "not bothersome" now and caused no trouble, the staff gave her a "female honor card," permitting her to walk around the hospital grounds.

On July 18, 1968, she was discharged. Returning to New York City, she discovered that all her property had disappeared from the King Edward Hotel. The list was short: "one canvas bag, two coats, clothing in closet, bag of canned food, one suitcase, various cosmetics and property in vanity drawers, etc."; but it was all she had, and it was gone. Two property agents from the Department of Mental Hygiene contacted the hotel and received the standard reply: "Manager informed us that someone broke into the baggage room and everything in there was stolen."

Mary Summers tried to piece her life together, but in addition to her other problems, she now lived under the constant apprehension that she would be carted off to the hospital for the slightest misstep. Her memories and fears drove her deeper into herself, her room, her constricted world. Gradually, fear gave way to anger and withdrawal to outrage. On June 18, 1969, exactly one year after her conversion to voluntary status, she called me.

It took me only a moment to realize that Miss Summers was no ordinary complainant. Her narrative was precise, intelligent, and frequently eloquent. While she was testy and easily provoked to anger when recalling her experiences, she freely admitted the eccentricity of her life style. My chief impression of her then (and now) was of a person with a precise sense of herself.

Furthermore, I was interested enough in the facts of her commitment and the constitutionality of the statutes under which she had been committed to join her as a plaintiff in a lawsuit I had already filed (see chapter twelve). But I was even more interested in what had happened to her after she was hospitalized —interested enough to begin a new lawsuit, which proceeded on the assumption that even if she had been lawfully hospitalized (a point we disputed in the other case), she still had certain constitutional rights that went with her into the hospital. To have subjected her to forced medication, photographing, and fingerprinting was, we alleged, a violation of those rights.

The case was assigned, by lot, to Federal Judge Anthony J. Travia, a recent appointment. On the surface this was a hopeful development. Judge Travia had been Speaker of the Assembly of the New York legislature when it voted to repeal the statute requiring the photographing and fingerprinting of mental patients, and later when it voted to make the requirement permissive rather than mandatory (Governor Nelson Rockefeller had vetoed both bills). Judge Travia, however, had also been Speaker in 1964, when the legislature enacted the sections of the mental hygiene law under which Mary Summers had been hospitalized. I tried to size him up as he went through the calendar. He was hard-nosed, no doubt about that, and accustomed to exercising power, to giving orders.

Eventually the clerk called *Summers* v. *Miller.** I argued for almost an hour before Judge Travia and left the courtroom confident. But when the decision came, it was a disaster.

---

* Alan D. Miller, M.D., was the commissioner of the Department of Mental Hygiene. In this position, he became a necessary defendant in any broad-scale attack on the mental hygiene laws; the directors of Bellevue and Central Islip were joined as additional defendants.

The law says that *sane* people have the right to refuse medication on religious grounds. If Mary Summers had been a patient
in a general rather than a mental hospital, the doctors would not
have dared to inject her with medication over her protest; if they
had, she could have sued the hospital for assault and battery,
and won. I had argued that her presence in a mental hospital did
not mean she was mentally ill—after all, no court had ever found
her to be mentally ill—and she should therefore have had the
same rights as a patient in a general hospital. But Judge Travia,
pointing out that she "could summarily have been found to be an
incompetent," decided to treat her as if she *had* been found by a
court to be incompetent, ignoring the fact that if she had received a court hearing, the court might well have pronounced her
sane and ordered her discharged.

I had also argued that there was no emergency—her life was
not in danger—and thus no reason to begin medication without
court authorization. Even if there was some justification for beginning the medication without judicial approval—and I could
think of none—there was certainly no justification for continuing
the medication for three months without once asking a court to
resolve the dispute. To that argument, Judge Travia answered
(irrelevantly, I thought) that the doctors had acted in "good
faith."

My main argument, however, had been that followers of Christian Science believe it is wrong to accept medical treatment of a
physical nature (a point the judge conceded), so that even if
Miss Summers had been, in the doctors' view, mentally competent, she would still have refused medication on religious
grounds. In other words, her mental competence, or lack of it,
was irrelevant. About that, the judge said nothing at all.

Judge Travia dismissed Mary Summers's objection to the photographing and fingerprinting as "obviously without merit" and
"insubstantial." Why? Because of what hospital officials "might"
have done with that information; it "might be useful in identify-

ing a patient" whose identity is not known, or in "aiding in determining if a patient had previously been treated in a state mental institution." He did not think it important that the hospital certainly knew who Miss Summers was and knew—as was noted in its records—that this was "her first admission to a mental hospital." He did not care that photos and prints are almost never used for these purposes; that was why the legislature, at the recommendation of the Department of Mental Hygiene, had voted to relax the requirement. Perhaps the taking of her prints did not, as we thought, substantially invade Miss Summers's right of privacy. But certainly the forwarding of those prints to the New York State Identification and Intelligence System raised serious issues. Mary Summers would never know who had been told of her hospitalization, and she would have no opportunity to rebut the stigma of criminality or mental illness that the existence of those records conveys. That, it seemed to us, was an unnecessary abridgment of her constitutional "right to be let alone," as Justice Louis Brandeis once phrased it. Judge Travia disagreed.

With the help of William Pratt, the attorney who had volunteered to help in the Long case, I began piecing together a detailed appellate brief, which eventually ran to more than a hundred pages.

Our strategy on appeal was quite different from our strategy in the lower court. After studying Judge Travia's opinion, I began to sense the hidden premise of his decision: if Mary Summers was crazy enough to be hospitalized against her will, she was too crazy to decide for herself whether to accept or reject tranquilizing medication. The judge had held, in effect, that once you are lawfully hospitalized, the doctors can do whatever they want to you, so long as they act in good faith. In other words, the judge had not accepted our premise that the legality of what happens to a person *after* hospitalization is a question separate from the legality of the process by which he is brought *to* the hospital. Even under this reasoning, however, it should follow that if Mary

Summers was well enough to leave, she was well enough to decide the type of treatment she would accept if she stayed.

In the lower court, I had argued that Miss Summers was an involuntary patient who had been converted to voluntary status under duress; on appeal, we said not a word about duress. We simply pointed out that she was, for one month, a voluntary patient, and thus presumably competent to accept or reject hospitalization. Furthermore, the Central Islip records indicated quite clearly that on May 15, 1968, long before her conversion to voluntary status, Mary Summers had understood what was going on around her.

ORIENTATION: Well as to the three spheres. [This means she was normal with respect to her understanding of time, place, and person.]

RECENT MEMORY: Good.

RETENTION AND RECALL: Good.

COUNTING AND CALCULATIONS: Good.

SCHOOL AND GENERAL KNOWLEDGE: Good.

ABSTRACTION ABILITY: Good.

JUDGMENT: Normal.

And yet, on the day of that entry and every day thereafter, Mary Summers was forced to take medication over her continuing objections. Central Islip's doctors did not think she was a raving lunatic; to the contrary, they thought her judgment normal. Why, then, did they not respect her judgment? Apparently because of the following cryptic statement contained in the same mental status report: "Insight: More impaired on personal matters than on impersonal matters." The meaning of that statement is explained in the summary of the mental status report, which notes that she was "holding a Bible in her hands . . . patient stated that she is a Christian Scientist. She showed religious preoccupations and mild feelings of persecution." The thread that runs through almost every page of the Bellevue and Central Islip records—in fact, the only thing about Mary Summers that was not normal—was her "preoccupation" with religion. Even her mild feelings of persecution stemmed directly from that preoccupation. Furthermore, by June 18, 1968, Central Islip believed her insight, even with respect to personal matters, had improved sufficiently to justify conversion from involuntary to voluntary status.

We would hammer that point home again and again: if Mary Summers was well enough to decide whether she should be in the hospital at all, why wasn't she well enough to decide whether to accept or reject medication? The defendants never came up with an answer.

Our new strategy worked. On May 26, 1971, almost eight months after the appeal had been argued, a three-judge panel of the Second Circuit Court of Appeals, one of the most prestigious courts in the nation, reversed Judge Travia by ruling that mental patients do have a constitutional right to refuse medication on religious grounds.

The decision was extremely important, for it made possible a series of new challenges to the mental hospital system. In the past, most of the important cases involving mental patients had challenged the commitment process, without questioning what happened after hospitalization. The Summers case and the others I have just described in part II are among a handful demonstrating that even lawfully hospitalized persons retain constitutional rights, which must be respected.

Hospital administrators do not like the new and uncomfortable feeling of federal judges looking over their shoulders, so it was not surprising when the defendants appealed the Second Circuit's decision to the United States Supreme Court. They knew that if the decision stood, there would soon be other challenges to what goes on inside mental hospitals. Cases would arise challenging censorship of patients' mail and restrictions on their rights to receive visitors, to be examined by outside psychiatrists of their choosing, to wear their own clothes instead of hospital uniforms, and to have more fresh air and exercise. The issues are many. In fact, hospital administrators became so alarmed that the Hospital Association of New York State joined in the appeal and asked the Supreme Court to reverse the Second Circuit Court of Appeals, claiming that if the decision were permitted to stand, it would "wreak havoc" with the mental hospital system, as indeed it would.

On December 7, 1971, the Supreme Court announced that it would let the decision of the Second Circuit stand. Ahead of us still was an argument before Judge Travia to collect monetary damages for Mary Summers. That would be a hard, time-consuming trial. But we had established a new legal principle. The locked doors of mental hospitals everywhere had been opened, a little, to let the Constitution in.

Part III
One-Way Street

The doctor is often more to be feared than the disease.

If two doctors say "this man is mad," they will be believed. If later they say "now he is sane," they will not be believed. In the public mind, mental illness is irreversible: once mad, always mad, or close to it.

In the job market, it is better to be an ex-convict than an ex-mental patient. Many employers are willing to say of the ex-convict that "he has paid his debt to society," but very few employers will knowingly hire an ex-mental patient. Almost all public employers and most large companies ask job applicants if they have ever been hospitalized for mental illness. If the answer is yes, the applicant will almost certainly not get the job; if the applicant lies and says no, he runs the risk of eventual discovery through state fingerprint files and other records.

It is time for psychiatrists and judges to face the brutal facts. When they commit a person to a mental hospital, they are taking away not only his liberty, but also any chance he might have for a decent life in the future.

Even voluntary hospitalization creates so many problems and closes so many doors that an old joke takes on new truth—a person has to be crazy to sign himself into a mental hospital.

9 / Stigma I

The year 1949 was a bad one for thirteen-year-old Henry Alexander Mercer. His mother died suddenly of a heart attack, terminating the modest family income and leaving Henry to the erratic care of an alcoholic father. His father cursed Henry when drunk and beat him when sober, once with a leather belt and once by tying his hands behind his back and pushing him into a tub of water, from which his half sisters rescued him. Henry was pretty much on his own—if he wanted a decent meal, he had to cook it himself; if he needed a winter coat, he either had to steal it or go cold. And so he began to steal, and lie, and cheat.

Henry was an exceedingly bright boy. When he had the time

and energy, which was not often, he read Plato and Emerson, fascinated by them even at his age. But school was not as important as survival, which dictated an impossibly hard schedule for one so young. Henry frequently worked until one or two in the morning as an unlicensed porter in the Port Authority Bus Terminal in Manhattan, and was out before dawn delivering newspapers. He was often late to school or absent from class. When he was there, he usually sat slumped behind his desk, bruised and scratched from some street-corner brawl of the night before, or fell asleep.

Teachers began to ask him what was wrong, but Henry was proud, and not about to tell them that his family life had collapsed. If they persisted, they were told to mind their own business. Several times he threw erasers at teachers who would not let him alone, and more than once his outbursts completely disrupted a class.

The police were beginning to compile a file on Henry Mercer. Nothing serious—stealing an apple from a fruit stand, hanging around pool halls—but clearly, at the rate he was going, Henry Mercer would soon graduate to bigger trouble.

No doubt about it, Henry was a problem. His teachers could not handle him, his father would not, and no one else cared. He had not yet done anything to justify a jail sentence or reform school, but he had to be put somewhere, or so the authorities thought. Therefore, on February 17, 1949, with his father's consent, Henry Mercer was committed to Rockland State Mental Hospital, his home for the next four years.

The doctors knew almost from the start that Henry did not belong there. His diagnosis ("primary behavior disorder in children—conduct disturbance") was reserved for children who were unruly but definitely not psychotic. Almost immediately, "he was considered well enough to leave the hospital." Yet because of his father's antagonism, he could not be sent home, and the hospital's repeated attempts to find a foster home were unsuccessful. (According to state legislators and family court judges, there were almost 600 other children at Rockland State more or less like Henry Mercer. They were not criminals nor were they crazy. They were lonely kids from broken homes, for whom society could provide nothing better than a mental hospital.)

Little worth remembering happened during Henry's four years at Rockland State. His father visited him once, and, finally, so did his older brother, Jack, just out of the Marine Corps. When Jack was told by the supervising psychiatrist that there was "nothing wrong" with his brother, he agreed to look after Henry, who was immediately discharged to his custody.

Henry was now seventeen. After his discharge, he worked as a laborer until he took up boxing, eventually doing well enough to appear in Madison Square Garden and even sparring occasionally with Floyd Patterson. In the spring and summer he played semiprofessional baseball. In 1959, after four years of night school, he earned a high school diploma.

Henry Mercer settled down to work as a nurse's aide at Lincoln Hospital in the Bronx and did so well that in 1965—the year he married—he was promoted to ambulance attendant. The work was demanding and full of excitement. Each call brought a new emergency—he delivered babies, administered heart massage and mouth-to-mouth resuscitation, put splints on broken bones, and patched up knife wounds. Many of his "calls" were drunk or violent (twice he was punched in the face), but Mercer never lost his temper. It was not long before he was assigned to the "out-bus," an ambulance reserved for the most difficult calls.

In 1968, he learned that his second child was on the way. Although this pleased the Mercers, it also meant that Henry would have to pick up extra money on nights and weekends. In New York City, one of the best ways to do that is to drive a cab.

In December, 1968, Mercer took the subway to the Hack License Bureau, paid the five-dollar fee, filled out an application, passed the geography test, and stood in line waiting for his medical exam. When he entered the examination room, the doctor took one look at his application form and threw up his hands.

"It says here that you have been hospitalized for a nervous or mental condition. Is that right?"

"Yes sir, in 1949."

"Was that a mental hospital?"

"Yes, Rockland State."

"Then you might as well get out of here, because we can't give you a license."

"Why not?"

"Because you have been in a mental hospital, that's why."

"But there's nothing wrong with me now, and I can prove it. Look, I've got a letter from the director of Rockland State and from another psychiatrist, and both of them say there's no reason why I shouldn't be driving a cab."

"I don't care what your letters say. I don't even want to see them. It doesn't make any difference. You've been a mental patient and that means you can't get a license. If you want to appeal, you'll have to take it up with Dr. McCoy, the chief police surgeon. Now I really can't spend any more time with you. I've got other people to see. Sorry, but that's the rule."

Mercer sent his two letters to Dr. McCoy and offered to submit to a new psychiatric examination by Hack Bureau psychiatrists. Three months later McCoy's office declined this offer and told Mercer that "no further consideration can be taken on your application." That was when he came to see me.

Henry Mercer is muscular, athletic, and handsome. When off duty, he usually wears chinos, a brightly colored polo shirt, and a black felt, Indian-style hat—as a black man, he relates to the Indians' oppression and pride. Occasionally he dons a brightly patterned dashiki made by his wife. Mercer talks easily about the things that interest him—about good food (he is a health-food enthusiast) and keeping in shape (he jogs at least one mile, and frequently five or six, in Central Park every day). And about religion: "Religion is a lot of junk. There's only one Jesus and one

Buddha, and they both did the same thing. I never go to church and my children won't go either. I wouldn't let the priest baptize my child. He thought I was crazy. I've seen what the church does. My uncle was a Baptist minister. When I got out of Rockland, he said, 'You're on your own now.' He died a few months ago, and everyone at the funeral talked about how he helped the poor. But he never helped his own nephew."

It did not take me long to draft a complaint and rough out a brief. In 1964, the New York legislature had passed a statute designed to eliminate per se discrimination against former voluntary mental patients:

Notwithstanding any other provision of law to the contrary no person admitted to a hospital by voluntary or informal admission shall be deprived of any civil right solely by reason of such admission nor shall such admission modify or vary any civil right of any such person, including but not limited to civil service ranking and appointment or rights relating to the granting, forfeiture or denial of a license, permit, privilege or benefit pursuant to any law.

Although Mercer had not been a voluntary patient in the strictest sense, he had been hospitalized as a minor upon the voluntary application of his father, and his admission was therefore at least arguably within the meaning of the statute. Certainly he had been denied a license solely because of his former status as a patient.

In mid-April, I filed what is called an Article 78 petition against Howard R. Leary, the Police Commissioner of the City of New York (the Police Department oversees the Hack Bureau), Louis M. Neco, deputy commissioner in charge of licenses, and Stephen M. McCoy, M.D., the chief surgeon of the department. The corporation counsel, the legal representative for all city employees, requested a week's adjournment, and then another. Finally, on May 29, I appeared in court with Mercer, who had brought along his four-year-old son.

We were number 151 on the calendar. After the clerk had

gone through the "first call" to record defaults and uncontested adjournments, Judge Amos Bowman entered from his robing room and stepped up to the bench to handle the second call. Mercer and I were encouraged to see that he was black.

I told Judge Bowman that the Hack Bureau had a firm policy of rejecting former mental patients, no matter how stable their present mental condition. The corporation counsel adamantly insisted this was not so. "Why, just this week the Hack Bureau granted a license to a former mental patient, a junior at Columbia University."

I was prepared for that. "Your Honor, I am amazed that the city can stand here and make that representation to you. I know the student they're talking about because I happen to be his lawyer, too. He applied for a license and they turned him down cold. It was only after I threatened to sue on his behalf, and after I filed this suit, that they gave him a license, apparently so they could come in here and claim they don't discriminate against former patients."

Bowman could see things might get messy. Wanting to avoid that, he turned to the corporation counsel.

"Look, this man is already working for a city hospital. He's already an ambulance attendant. Why shouldn't he drive a cab?"

"Well, Your Honor, that decision is made by the chief surgeon of the Police Department, whose duty it is by law to protect the public from—"

"I know, but if he reapplies, he'll get the license, won't he?"

"That's not my decision, Your Honor."

"Well," Bowman said, turning to me, "why don't you just reapply and see if you get it this time? If you don't, you can come back to court."

I was against that course. "Your Honor, I don't see why we should reapply. This is an open-and-shut case. The Hack Bureau rejected Mr. Mercer without any regard for his current mental condition, and that rejection is directly prohibited by statute. At the very least, this court should set aside that rejection as unlawful, and then remand the case to the Hack Bureau for further consideration."

"Well, I don't see any reason to get into all that. I'm sure that if you reapply, they will give the application serious consideration."

And that was that. No decision, no precedent, not even a mild rebuke to the Hack Bureau from the court. Mercer was right back where he had started almost six months earlier.

The first round had been an eye opener. I had not known what "arbitrary and capricious" meant until I read the Hack Bureau's answer to Mercer's complaint. The answer admitted that since 1959 it had been the written policy of the Hack Bureau that "candidates for hack driver's license whose investigation or findings reveal the presence or history of hospitalization or treatment for neurological or mental disorder are to be disqualified for hack driver's license." And Dr. McCoy confirmed that the 1959 policy had "essentially been continued." He claimed, however, that there had been a "modification" under which "if evidence is submitted on behalf of the applicant [that] there is no reasonable probability that the mental condition which caused the hospitalization of the applicant would occur again under stress situations, then the applicant would qualify for a hack driver's license."

The modification, if it existed, was present only in the mind of Dr. McCoy. He had not bothered to reduce it to writing, or to communicate it to his subordinates, who were still busily rejecting applicants on the basis of the 1959 rule. Even more important, however, was the type of evidence McCoy would require before granting a license. Mercer had supplied letters from Dr. Alfred M. Stanley, director of Rockland State Hospital, and from Dr. David E. Lehine, medical director of the Queens County Psychiatric Institute. McCoy ignored both.

Dr. Alfred Stanley, director of Rockland State Hospital, in his letter of February 3, 1969, says that in his opinion, Henry Mercer has "recovered sufficiently"—not recovered, just in Dr. Stanley's opinion "sufficiently". . . [he] does not state that in his opinion Mr. Mercer should be given a hack driver's license, just a license to operate a motor vehicle.

In his typewritten letter, Dr. Stanley had said that Mercer was a "suitable person to make application for a license to operate a motor vehicle." In his own handwriting, he had added "or to have a hack license," followed by his signature. McCoy had disregarded the handwritten notation, because it did not serve his purpose, and asserted boldly that Dr. Stanley approved Mercer only for a regular license, not a hack license.

McCoy gave even shorter shrift to Dr. Lehine's letter, dated December 19, 1968, which concluded that there was "no contraindication at the present time" why Mercer should not drive a cab. According to McCoy, the words "present time" meant that "Dr. Lehine's opinion, therefore, no longer holds for 12:01 A.M. on December 19, 1968 or any time subsequent."

That was a truly remarkable statement. In McCoy's view, Dr. Lehine's opinion that Mercer was competent to drive a cab retained its medical significance for only one day, yet Mercer's hospitalization, which had terminated almost two decades earlier, was not only medically significant but virtually conclusive.

McCoy's disdain for the expert opinion of two disinterested psychiatrists, who did not receive a penny for their efforts, was consistent with his apparent belief that mental illness can never be cured. In a conversation with a lawyer acquaintance of mine, McCoy had explained that he would issue hack licenses to former patients "if we could establish that their hospital records showed no findings of mental illness." In other words, evidence that nothing was currently wrong with an applicant would not suffice. McCoy had to be shown that the applicant's hospitalization had been a mistake.

Given McCoy's obvious prejudice against former patients, he

clearly would not give Mercer a license unless his reapplication was overwhelmingly strong. We set about making the case. Doctors Stanley and Lehine supplied more-detailed letters and affidavits, Mercer and his brother prepared affidavits to describe the circumstances of his hospitalization and his work record since discharge, and the assistant hospital administrator at Lincoln Hospital attested to Mercer's excellent work record. We capped off the reapplication with a three-page report signed jointly by four more psychiatrists, who agreed that there was absolutely nothing wrong with Mercer.

His mental status examination revealed no disorder. He was co-operative and demonstrated good judgment and insight.

It is our opinion that Mr. Mercer's behavioral disorder was of a transient nature and that he has demonstrated a definite and constant trend in successful mastery of his impulses since leaving the hospital. There is absolutely no indication that there will be any reoccurrence of the type of behavior that was manifest when Mr. Mercer was 13 years old and there is no indication at this time that he will be more prone than the average adult to mental illness in the future.

Furthermore, after wading through his hospital record, the psychiatrists were able to report that "he at no time demonstrated any psychotic behavior while in the hospital." In short, he was not crazy then or now, and was not likely to be in the future.

On June 18, 1969, we sent these papers to the Hack Bureau and requested reconsideration. On June 26, I wrote Dr. McCoy requesting either a decision or a date by which he intended to reach a decision. No reply. I wrote again on July 2. Still no reply. Finally I telephoned. McCoy's only reaction to our evidence was that it was "unfair" of Mercer to obtain favorable psychiatric evaluations from "his friends at Lincoln Hospital." I assured McCoy that although four of the psychiatrists did work at Lincoln, they had never met Mercer prior to their examination. McCoy said he had decided upon a date by which he would reach a decision, but he refused to tell me what that date was. Subsequent conversations with the assistant corporation counsel convinced me the city was stalling and would sit on the application for months to come. We had no choice but to return to court.

Normally, an Article 78 proceeding (a special proceeding against a public officer) is instituted by filing a petition, which the other side is given twenty days to answer. But the Hack Bureau was already so familiar with this case that it wouldn't need twenty days. I therefore began the second court round by obtaining an order to show cause, signed by a judge, which expressly incorporated by reference the petition used in round one, and which gave the Hack Bureau only five days, until August 4, to answer. The bureau countered by filing a motion to strike the whole case from the calendar on the ground that we had not filed a new petition in round two. The motion was frivolous, raised only to forestall a decision on the merits. Still, it meant I had to prepare opposing papers and a memorandum of law and trudge down to court, wasting yet another day. On September 11, the judge dismissed the Hack Bureau's motion and gave the bureau ten days to reach a decision.

At that point, McCoy, who is not a psychiatrist, contended that he could not properly evaluate the unanimous opinion of the six psychiatrists who had examined Mercer until he had personally studied Mercer's hospital record. McCoy also claimed that the opinions expressed in the joint report were "not statistically valid" because they were "based on a short interview without psycnological testing." McCoy, of course, had reached a contrary opinion without any interview or testing. I could not help wondering whether he would have questioned the statistical validity of the joint report if the four psychiatrists had agreed with him.

McCoy's insistence on reviewing the hospital record was, in

my view, disingenuous. When Mercer initially applied for a license, he had signed a release authorizing McCoy to request a copy of his record, but McCoy had not bothered to do so. Six months later, Mercer had signed another release. Did McCoy really expect to find damaging evidence buried in twenty-year-old records, evidence that had somehow escaped the attention of the five psychiatrists who had already examined them? Rockland State had, in fact, sent McCoy a six-page clinical summary of the hospital record, though he claimed he had not received it. And so it went. Nothing to do but return to court for round three.

There, I practically begged Judge Jacob Grumet to render a decision on the merits, but, like Judge Bowman, he wanted no part of it. He commented that the Hack Bureau had not received the full hospital record, which I considered irrelevant.

Your Honor, five psychiatrists have already reviewed those records and have found nothing damaging in them. Certainly respondent McCoy, who is not even a psychiatrist, is in no position to second-guess their collective judgment. But if there were something damaging in those records, and there is not, it would relate only to Mr. Mercer's mental condition twenty years ago, not today. As we have shown in our briefs, the mental hygiene law absolutely prohibits discrimination against former mental patients when the only basis for the discrimination is their *past* mental condition. There is not one shred of evidence that there is anything wrong with Mr. Mercer now, or likely to be in the future. Quite the contrary. Thus, if the Hack Bureau disapproved his application based on something they found in his records, they would be in direct violation of the statute. Accordingly, since the records can't possibly serve as a legitimate basis for denying Mr. Mercer's application, there is no reason to adjourn this proceeding yet another time.

But there was reason enough for Grumet, who adjourned the case until October 30, when a fourth judge would have to worry about it. Dejectedly, I began to prepare for round four.

By then, however, the Hack Bureau had begun to see that although the decision could be delayed for perhaps a few months, sooner or later some judge would be forced to rule on the merits; and when he did, the Hack Bureau was bound to lose. On October 21, the bureau offered to settle the case. It would give Mercer his license if he dropped the suit and agreed to furnish psychiatric evaluations at six-month intervals. I was tempted not to pass the offer on to Mercer—if he accepted, months of work would go down the drain, and there would be no decision others could rely upon. But I forced myself to call him and explain the details. He asked my advice.

"Well, Mr. Mercer, to be perfectly frank, if I were you I would accept the settlement."

"But then we wouldn't get a decision, would we?"

"No."

"Then maybe we better just go on like we are."

"Well, of course, I would prefer to get a decision, because I think we would win. But you can never be sure with litigation, and the settlement is a certainty. Besides, even if we won they could appeal and delay the final decision for months. Even if we won on appeal, you might not get your license for a year or more."

Mercer needed the license now. The addition of a baby daughter had stretched an already slim paycheck to the breaking point. So we settled.*

On the day Mercer picked up his license we had a brief celebration in my office, featuring a three-layer chocolate cake his wife had made entirely from organic ingredients. Mercer expressed confidence about his future. By working as an ambulance attendant at night and driving a cab days and weekends, he thought he would be able to make it. It would not be an easy

---

* Two years later, because of Mercer's unblemished record, we convinced the Hack Bureau to drop the periodic evaluation requirement.

life, but he did not mind hard work. All he had wanted was a chance, and now he had it.

Mercer's troubles were not over, though. The following day, the New York *Post* and the *Times* carried stories about his year-long struggle with the Hack Bureau, and word got around that "Henry Mercer is a former mental patient." Overnight, his expectations began to crumble—even a few of the ambulance drivers who had worked with him for years refused to accompany him on calls now that they knew the "truth," and former friends avoided him.

Two weeks later, on November 22, 1969, at 11:00 P.M., Louis Andrews telephoned Lincoln Hospital and requested emergency assistance for his wife, Nancy. Mercer grabbed his medical bag and jumped into an ambulance driven by John A. Alexander. Racing up the stairs to the Andrews apartment, he found the patient lying on the floor, conscious but dizzy, surrounded by her husband and two patrolmen. Mercer asked them to stand back and give her some air. The cops told Mercer to get a wheelchair. Mercer said he didn't have a wheelchair and that they would have to use a stretcher. The cops said a stretcher wouldn't work, Mercer said it would, and one of the cops said, "How would you know? You're stinking drunk." Mercer said that wasn't true and turned to the patient. The cops ordered him to leave the apartment and radio for another attendant, which he did.

Two months later, Mercer received a notice to report to the Department of Hospitals for a disciplinary hearing. He was charged with leaving the premises "with a total disregard for the comfort and safety of the patient," and with "negligence in leaving the carry chair in the emergency room." If he lost the hearing, he could lose his job. Even suspension for a few days would mean that his pending application for promotion to ambulance driver would automatically be denied.

The charge did not make sense to me. First, I was sure Mercer had not been drunk—he rarely drank at all. And he had been on duty for almost eight hours, constantly observed, too busy even to sit down. Second, it is the responsibility of the ambulance driver, not the attendant, to see that a wheelchair is in the ambulance. Strangest of all was the fact that Police Commissioner Howard R. Leary, a defendant in Mercer's action against the Hack Bureau, had written to the Department of Hospitals requesting the disciplinary hearing. The two patrolmen admitted that incidents as trivial as this were not normally reported to Leary. It seemed likely that word had gone down to get Mercer.

We obtained affidavits from the patient and her husband, from the ambulance driver, and from Theodore B. Bonnemere, the ambulance dispatcher at Lincoln. All agreed that Mercer "was not drunk or in any way under the influence of alcohol." At the hearing, the cops denied having ordered Mercer to leave, but the patient, her husband, and the driver all specifically recalled hearing the order. Bonnemere and Alexander explained the absence of the wheelchair: after the previous call, the doctor on duty in the emergency ward, which was already crowded beyond capacity, had ordered Mercer and Alexander to "leave the ambulance wheelchair on the ward, as there was no other place to seat the patient." Louis Andrews reported that "at all times while Mr. Mercer was present in the apartment, he was very courteous and helpful to my wife and, in my opinion, he did all that he could to act in her interest. He was very considerate of her comfort and safety." His wife agreed. "I recall that I was lying on the floor and Mr. Mercer was bending over me. He said, 'Everything's going to be all right. Don't worry.' . . . While Mr. Mercer was with me, he was at all times respectful and considerate of my welfare. His behavior was in no way objectionable."

At the conclusion of the hearing, the hearing officer commented that he had decided beforehand to suspend Mercer for fifteen days, but now, because of "conflicting testimony of the people involved," he was going to limit the suspension to three days.

I demanded to speak to the hearing officer in private. After the room had been cleared, I reviewed the evidence and asked how he could possibly rule against Mercer. He admitted that there was very little evidence against him, but, after all, two police officers had taken the time and trouble to show up for the hearing, and it would be an "insult" to them (or to Leary?) if Mercer were exonerated. I pointed out that even a one-hour suspension would mean Mercer could never become an ambulance driver or hold down any other civil service job. Finally, he agreed to reverse his decision. Everyone was reassembled and the hearing officer announced that he had "changed his mind." Instead of a suspension, Mercer would receive only a "written reprimand."

Three months later, Mercer was promoted to ambulance driver. He survived the six-month probationary period without incident and was granted civil service tenure.

10 / Stigma II

Henry Mercer got his hack license and, ultimately, civil service ranking as an ambulance driver; others like him did not. In the week following the newspaper acounts of his settlement with the Hack License Bureau, twenty-three persons called to report that they too had been denied hack licenses because of a history of psychiatric disorder. Most of them had never been hospitalized; it was enough that their selective service records indicated they had been classified 1Y or 4F (unacceptable) because of "emotional" or "character" problems. All had gone to the Hack Bureau with letters from psychiatrists who said there was nothing currently wrong with them. I started a class action naming seven of the twenty-three as representatives of all applicants who had been denied hack licenses solely because of their past.

The Hack Bureau refused to answer the complaint or submit to depositions. The bureau initiated settlement discussions and then, after three months of negotiation, broke them off. More than a year after the case was filed, we still had no decision on the merits.

There was also the case of Nicholas Martinez. The New York City Civil Service Commission had successively denied his applications for jobs as trackman for the New York City Transit Authority, patrolman for the New York City Transit Police, housing patrolman for city housing projects, patrolman for the Police Department, railroad clerk, sanitation man, and correction officer. His scores on the written examinations ranged from a low of 77 per cent to a high of 92 per cent. Each time the commission turned him down because several years before he had been a voluntary patient in a state mental hospital for eight months. With each application he had submitted current psychiatric reports stating there was nothing wrong with him, or had offered to submit to examination by commission psychiatrists. The following rejection letter, quoted in full, is illustrative:

You were marked not qualified by our psychiatrist because your case history indicated that you were hospitalized at Central Islip State Hospital. This disqualification is in accordance with the medical standards. Any psychiatric examination would be a waste of time.

I lost his case on procedural grounds—all the applications had been denied more than four months before he came to see me, and our action was therefore barred by a special rule that requires persons who feel aggrieved by New York City agencies to sue within four months of the incident. There is an exception to that rule— the "continuing wrong" exception—which the court could have cited if it had wanted to help Nicholas Martinez; but it did not.

He tried again, taking and passing (with an adjusted final average of 97 per cent) all tests necessary to become a bridge and tunnel officer—a toll collector on the George Washington Bridge or in the Lincoln or Hudson Tunnel. This time, the Civil Service Commission was more politic; instead of denying his application on psychiatric grounds, which we would have challenged within the required four months, it did nothing. More than a year later, Nicholas Martinez had been neither accepted nor rejected, despite repeated requests for a decision.

Over the years I have made similar charges of per se discrimination against the Welfare Department, the Board of Education, and other city and state agencies. Some of my clients have won; most of them have lost. But none was able to force a case through to a judicial decision on the merits. None, that is, except an extraordinary young woman named Myra Lee Glassman.

Myra graduated *magna cum laude* from the City College of New York (CCNY), made Phi Beta Kappa in her junior year, and had been in the CCNY honors program in both chemistry and psychology. Her list of awards also included a Regents College Scholarship, granted by the state of New York to exceptional graduates of the state's high schools, and a National Science Foundation grant for research in chemistry. In the fall of the academic year 1968–69, after scoring in the top 1 per cent in science and quantitative ability on the nationwide Medical College Admission Test, she applied for admission to thirteen medical schools. She was rejected by every one. She wasn't told why, but she knew. Two years earlier, between her sophomore and junior years, she had spent a year as a voluntary patient at Hillside Hospital, one of the better private psychiatric facilities in the United States. Each medical school had questioned her about that, and it was clear from the questions that they were not willing to take a risk on a former mental patient.

As she described her experiences, I tried to determine what

kind of witness she would make. She was twenty-four, attractive, with long dark hair and a tidy, freshly scrubbed appearance. A miniskirt dispelled what might otherwise have seemed a somewhat prim demeanor. She was confident and highly verbal, precise in her answers, and not at all crazy. All in all, an unusually sympathetic witness.

Myra Lee Glassman never would have been a mental patient if her parents had raised her to have any confidence in herself. A psychiatrist would later describe the source of her difficulties as "a sadistic, guilt-provoking, and dependent mother." Together, Myra's parents made her feel guilty even to be alive. Part of the problem was their strict religious orthodoxy.

They were Orthodox Jews and had raised Myra accordingly. She attended the Yeshiva of Flatbush, a Hebrew parochial high school, where she not only excelled in both Hebrew and secular subjects, but also participated actively in a variety of extracurricular activities, which gave her a creative outlet as well as a temporary escape from her intolerable family situation.

Gradually, however, Myra realized that while she identified strongly with her Hebrew cultural heritage, she could not accept Orthodox Judaism as her way of life. This independence of thought was something her parents refused to accept. To them, anything less than strict orthodoxy suggested grave moral shortcomings. Thus, religious arguments were added to their already rejecting and disparaging tirades against their daughter, who, they claimed, was worthless from the day she was born. As time went on, the rift between Myra's academic life and her personal life widened. Even after completing two years at CCNY with nearly a straight-A average, she could not escape "feelings of loneliness, low self-esteem, and just depression."

Later, she would testify that the "first step" toward self-sufficiency—to leave her parents' house, which they strongly opposed —had proved emotionally impossible. She blamed herself for her intolerable home life. She was sure she could "never make it" on her own—never be able to support herself, manage her own apartment, and continue school at the same time. A college psychiatrist had told her she was right in wanting to leave home. Yet she could not bring herself to do it. She therefore decided she would have to "manipulate the psychiatrist into deciding for me that I should enter a hospital, and the best way to do that would be to convince the psychiatrist, or people who had easy and free access to him, that I was about to commit suicide."

Several times she hinted at suicide, but the psychiatrist did not take her seriously. To make her threats more believable, she used her knowledge of chemistry to calculate the lethal dose of a common medication for a person of her body weight, and then took half that amount—enough to make her very sick, but not enough to kill her. Her parents and the psychiatrist still were not deceived. They didn't even pump her stomach.

In November of 1965, Myra Lee obtained some potassium thiocyanate, a nontoxic compound, showed it to a friend, and said she was on the way to the bus terminal to catch a bus for Philadelphia, where she intended to commit suicide. As she hoped, the friend called Myra's parents and told them, incorrectly, that Myra had some "cyanide," one of the most toxic of substances, and was going to take it. Two hours later, the police found her in the Port Authority Terminal calmly reading a book. Sure enough, she had in her purse two capsules of "cyanide," which the police confiscated (but never submitted for laboratory analysis).

Sergeant Johnson, the arresting officer, was less sanguine about her intentions than the psychiatrist had been. He took her to Montefiore Hospital for observation. And now that there had been a "crisis" which "proved" to her parents that she needed psychiatric help, Myra Lee at last felt able to make the break she had so long wanted. She left Montefiore and signed in as a voluntary patient at Hillside Hospital, where she would live for a little more than a year—a year during which her parents, who lived minutes away, would visit her only three times.

When Myra had finished her story, we decided to concentrate our efforts on New York Medical College, her last choice of the thirteen schools to which she had applied. It was, according to her, the least prestigious, and therefore the least able to claim that she had been rejected on academic grounds. The legal basis of our challenge was the same statute involved in Henry Mercer's case, Mental Hygiene Law Section 70, paragraph 5, which prohibited discrimination against former voluntary patients "solely" because they had been hospitalized, and protected their civil rights.

I knew from another New York statute, section 40 of the civil rights law, that the right to attend an "educational institution" was a "civil right" that could not be denied without good cause. I also knew from the mental hygiene law that the legislature had already determined that voluntary hospitalization alone did not constitute good cause.

I called (and later wrote) J. Frederick Eagle, the dean of New York Medical College, to inquire whether the college would voluntarily reconsider Miss Glassman's application, saving us the trouble, and the college the embarrassment, of litigation. I was careful to explain that we did not claim her past mental condition was irrelevant. To the contrary, I said, a medical school should consider whether applicants for admission are sufficiently stable to go through the admittedly difficult years of medical study. Past mental condition is certainly relevant to that consideration. Our claim, rather, was that past condition, while relevant to the future, is no *more* relevant than present condition. We contended that the college had a statutory duty to consider Miss Glassman's present mental condition before it attempted to predict her future. I was so certain that Myra had completely recovered from her past mental difficulties that I made the college an offer: she would submit to current psychiatric examinations and a review of her past history by any three psychiatrists the college chose to name; if any one of the three expressed the slightest doubt about her ability to succeed in medical school, we would drop the case. On the other hand, even if all three unanimously recommended that she be admitted, the college would not be bound by their recommendation; we would ask only that the college reconsider her application. The college declined our offer and we filed suit.

Our chances were slim. First, New York Medical College is a private institution, and it was unclear whether the statute prohibited discrimination by nongovernmental agencies. Second, even if the statute did apply, courts have generally been reluctant to interfere in the internal operations of educational institutions. Third, Myra Lee Glassman wanted to be a doctor. The social stigma that had made it impossible for Nicholas Martinez to sell tokens in a subway booth would be nothing compared with society's fear of entrusting lives to a former mental patient. Judges are human, and the prejudices I had discovered in the Hack Bureau and the Civil Service Commission were not likely to be absent from the courts.

The only real hope was a preliminary, or temporary, injunction, a court order that theoretically does nothing more than preserve the status quo pending a full-scale trial and decision on the merits. For example, if a timber company is threatening to cut down a sweep of giant redwoods along a federal highway, a conservation group might persuade a judge to order that no trees be cut until after the court has decided, through a trial, whether the company has the right to cut them; otherwise, by the time the case was tried the redwoods might be gone, and the court's final decision would be meaningless. In practice, however, the issuance of a preliminary injunction often ends the case; the party against whom the injunction is issued is likely to give up and never go to trial on the merits.

In September of 1969, I made a motion for a preliminary injunction, asking that the court order the college to permit Myra Lee to audit classes for the fall term so that she would not irreparably lose the time if the court ultimately decided, after trial, that she was entitled to be registered as a regular student. I believed she would do so well on her first-semester exams that the college would drop its opposition to her admission; at the least, good grades and a semester or two of successful study could only strengthen our position. I scheduled the motion before Judge Samuel A. Spiegel, who had shown himself to be an unusually courageous judge (in one recent case he had held unconstitutional many of the procedures governing the involuntary hospitalization of narcotics addicts). During oral argument, Judge Spiegel was visibly concerned with Myra Lee's plight, and he noted in his opinion that he had "explored the matter fully, for this bright young woman elicits compassion by her dilemma." Nevertheless, because the case raised such "serious" and far-reaching issues, he concluded, "reluctantly," that he was "constrained to deny this motion."

We had come close, but we had lost, and now we had to prepare for trial. The trial was held in a large courtroom on the fourth floor of the New York County Court House in lower Manhattan. There was no jury, because we were asking for "equitable" relief (admission to the college), and juries are permitted only when "legal" relief (monetary damages) is sought. The judge was Bernard Nadel, a short, pugnacious man, who let everyone know from the start that he was a no-nonsense judge. My cocounsel was Bernard D. Fischman, general counsel for the American Orthopsychiatric Association, an old and respected organization of psychiatrists, psychologists, and concerned laymen—the more liberal counterpart of the American Psychiatric Association. Fischman announced that "Ortho" wished to file an *amicus curiae*, friend-of-the-court, brief in support of Myra Lee's application for admission. The brief, prepared by Professor Alan Dershowitz of Harvard Law School and Dr. Alan Stone of Harvard Medical School, analyzed the undisputed facts and concluded that the college's rejection of Myra was unlawful and, more important, could not be justified on psychiatric grounds.*

Aside from Myra Lee Glassman, we had only one major witness, Dr. Joel S. Feiner, a young psychiatrist specializing in child and adolescent psychiatry. Feiner had graduated from Yale and, in 1964, from the Albert Einstein College of Medicine. Based on a personal examination of Myra, he "felt there was no reason at that time why—as a psychiatric opinion—she should not be admitted to medical school and why she could not fulfill the responsibilities of medical practice or medical education." He did not think she "represented either an emotional or an academic risk," and he characterized her past difficulties as "an adjustment reaction of adolescence," which "inevitably takes place" with adolescents, and was notable in her case only because it was "severe." The "situational" problem that prompted the reaction was without doubt her home environment; once she took up residence at Hillside and began to relate to persons other than her parents, the reaction had subsided.

At the time of his examination, some eight months after the college had rejected Myra Lee's application, he found absolutely no "evidence or symptoms of a current adjustment reaction or of any other mental disorder"; and he was able to state that her mental condition eight months earlier was probably equally healthy. In fact, the "serious stress" of the intervening rejection by thirteen medical schools would, if anything, have left her in worse mental condition at the time of his examination than at the time of her application, yet she had tolerated that stress

* The *amicus curiae* brief made three points: (1) the mere fact that a person has sought and received psychiatric treatment does not make such person more ill than persons who have not sought and received such treatment; (2) the mere fact that a student has sought and received psychiatric treatment in a mental hospital does not render such student a greater risk in terms of future academic achievement; (3) psychiatric screening is a particularly unreliable and inherently biased aspect of medical school admission procedures.

"quite well." Dr. Feiner thought the suicide threats were not bona fide attempts to commit suicide, but only "gestures" with "built-in safeguards," so that "never was she in danger from any of these."

Though Dr. Feiner was our only expert witness to appear in court, pursuant to an agreement with the other side I read into evidence the affidavits of several other persons.

Dr. Jonathan Cohen (whom I had met through Charlie Youngblood) had also examined Myra Glassman, and his written report, though prepared independently, was substantially identical to Dr. Feiner's testimony. He too was sure that "none" of the suicide threats "involved any serious or significant threat to her life." And he found "no evidence of any psychiatric condition which would impair her current or future functioning."

In applying to New York Medical College, Myra Lee had submitted three supporting recommendations by psychiatrists who had treated her in the past, including the clinical director of the adult inpatient services at Hillside, Dr. Richard S. Green. All three were intimately familiar with the circumstances of her hospitalization, and all had written letters that Dr. Feiner described as unqualifiedly "favorable" to her admission, a description the college did not dispute. Just before trial, Dr. Green examined Myra Lee again and submitted an affidavit pointing out that she was "better equipped to deal with the rigors of medical school than most other applicants" because she had "already succeeded" in coping with the stresses that are likely to affect everyone at some point in life. Thus, five psychiatrists were recommending her admission.

To that list of experts we added the affidavit of Nicholas Papouchis, a clinical psychologist on the staff of CCNY and a former teacher of Myra Lee's, who told the court he found "no evidence in her behavior that would indicate any difficulty handling the rigors of medical school training or the professional demands of medical practice. Her capacity to work independently, as indicated in the course of the semester, suggested, rather, that she would be an asset to any medical school." Other CCNY teachers, including Professors Neil McKelvie and Leonard H. Schwartz, considered her an "unusually mature, well-adjusted student" and saw no reason "to question her emotional stability."

Myra testified that after a month or two at Hillside she had begun to work twenty hours a week as a biochemistry research assistant for a Hillside doctor who had a grant to study drug metabolics and hormones. That had kept her busy for a while, but soon she began to miss the "academic challenge," so she had resumed classes at CCNY, earning A's in four-credit courses in comparative anatomy and honors economics—all the while returning to Hillside at night much as she would have returned to a hotel.

In the summer of 1967, she signed herself out of Hillside, got a job in a federal poverty program as a counselor for disturbed children, found a place to live, and earned two more A's in summer school. In the fall of 1967, living in her own apartment and supporting herself by working at the Jewish Guild for the Blind, she resumed full-time studies at CCNY and completed her last two years of college, improving on the almost perfect record she had compiled in the two years before she entered Hillside.

Shortly before graduation she had applied to New York Medical College. She was interviewed by Dr. Raymond McBride, a member of the admissions committee, whose report said:

Miss Glassman is a most impressive person. She was completely at ease and talked freely of her emotional problems. There is no doubt concerning her intellectual ability, and she appears to have genuine humanitarian motives behind her decision to enter medicine. I strongly recommend her acceptance. However, I feel that she should be interviewed by the psychiatrist because of her past history.

The psychiatrist chosen by New York Medical College was Dr. Benjamin Sadock, who was psychiatric consultant to the admissions committee. Up to this point, the application process had been perfectly straightforward, but we were never able to find out exactly what happened next. We knew that Dr. Sadock had recommended rejection of Miss Glassman's application, but we could not find out why. The official minutes of the admissions committee reveal that "Benjamin Sadock stated that we had accepted candidates who had recovered from mental illnesses, but that she had been rejected because of the nature of an ongoing illness." And at the beginning of the trial, the attorney for New York Medical College had contended that Myra Lee was rejected not because of her "past history," as Dr. McBride had put it, but because of "her condition at the time she was examined. That is our position." On cross-examination, however, Dr. Sadock denied telling the admissions committee that Myra Lee had an ongoing mental illness. He conceded that he "did not perform a classical or current mental status examination or make any current diagnosis." In fact, Dr. Sadock made no attempt to evaluate Myra Lee's current mental condition. He was interested only in her past. Yet his report to the other members of the admissions committee concluded: "Probable diagnosis of latent schizophrenia."

I pointed out to Dr. Sadock that the *Diagnostic and Statistical Manual* of the American Psychiatric Association limits the diagnosis of "latent schizophrenia" to persons "having clear symptoms of schizophrenia." Earlier in his testimony Dr. Sadock had admitted, reluctantly, that during the interview Miss Glassman appeared perfectly normal and did not exhibit "any withdrawn, regressive, or bizarre behavior." Obviously embarrassed about the flimsy basis for his diagnosis, Dr. Sadock requested an opportunity "to explain why I wrote that."

As I said, I did not do a history and mental status. I am not prepared

to say that Miss Glassman is schizophrenic. What I am prepared to
report to you is this fact, that most hospital admissions carry a diagnosis of schizophrenia. The majority of people who have been in
mental hospitals in a particular age group, her age group, have a
diagnosis of schizophrenia, and it was on that, sir, that I made that
comment. . . . I did not make that comment on the basis of a history
and a mental status. I am not prepared at this point to defend a diagnosis of schizophrenia in Miss Glassman. . . . I trust she does not
have that illness.

   With that admission, we proved more than I had thought we
could prove—no one at the college had conducted a current mental examination of Myra Lee Glassman. Dr. McBride had
strongly recommended that she be accepted, and had suggested
she see Dr. Sadock not because of any currently abnormal behavior, but only because of her past history. Dr. Sadock had told
the admissions committee he thought Myra was probably suffering from latent schizophrenia, but his report was based only on
his knowledge that she had been hospitalized, not on a current
examination.
   Clearly, her past history, and in particular her history of hospitalization, had figured prominently in her rejection. So the
college, remembering that the mental hygiene law did not pro-
hibit discrimination unless it was "solely" because of hospitalization, changed its position and claimed that she had been rejected
because of an "aggregate of factors," of which hospitalization
had been only one. Dr. Sadock testified that the so-called aggregate of factors included "her academic record, her scores on the
Medical College Admissions Test, the recommendations furnished by her, and the conclusions derived from personal interviews," and that no other major criteria were used. In advancing
his argument, Dr. Sadock specifically disagreed with the dean of
the college, who had written Myra Lee that she was in all respects a "well-qualified applicant" and was being rejected only
because of "the regrettable fact that there is not enough room."

In other words, Dr. Sadock said Miss Glassman was not qualified for admission under his aggregate of factors; Dean Eagle said she was qualified, though not as qualified as the 284 applicants whom the college accepted. I hoped to demonstrate that both positions were disingenuous by examining the aggregate of factors one by one.

First, Myra Lee's academic record was excellent. The college admitted that she was, so far as it knew, the only member of Phi Beta Kappa out of 2,870 applicants that year. Far from being academically unqualified, this would have made her the only Phi Beta Kappa in her entering class. Also, based on a state-wide test in which she placed twelfth, Myra Lee had been awarded a New York State Regents Medical Scholarship, given to college graduates who demonstrate exceptional promise for medical school. Fewer than 8 per cent of the applicants accepted by New York Medical College had won Regents Medical Scholarships.

Concerning the second of the aggregate factors, the scores on the Medical College Admissions Test, Dr. Sadock admitted that Myra Lee's put her within the upper 8 per cent of the accepted class, and that she may well have had the highest scores of any applicant—neither he nor anyone he had talked with knew of another applicant whose scores were as high or higher.

With respect to written recommendations, again Myra Lee promised to be an excellent medical student. She had submitted letters from three psychiatrists, each of whom, as we have seen, unqualifiedly favored her admission. The only other recommendation was an equally enthusiastic letter from the chairman of the recommendations committee of City College, which noted that Myra Lee's "emotional stability appears now to be very good," that she was "an excellent student" and "very reliable," that her "classroom participation was outstanding," and that she was considered by the entire recommendations committee to be "an excellent candidate for medical school." On cross-examination, Dr. Sadock first conceded that the CCNY letter was not "in and of itself" a basis for rejection, and then admitted that, to the contrary, "the letter of recommendation is good" and "would be considered a favorable letter."

It was clear, then, that Myra Lee Glassman's academic record, her MCAT scores, and her recommendations could not have been among the several factors that allegedly served as the basis for her rejection. The only other factor, according to Dr. Sadock, was the applicant's "motivation and promise for training and a career as a physician as revealed by the two personal interviews."

Dr. Sadock admitted that motivation alone was not a ground for rejecting Myra Lee's application; in fact, after interviewing her, both he and Dr. McBride "felt that she was well motivated." This left only her "promise" for a career as a doctor. Dr. McBride had no reservations on that score; he had "strongly recommended her acceptance." In the final analyis, Myra Lee was rejected not because of an aggregate of factors but because one man, Dr. Benjamin Sadock, disregarding the unanimous evidence to the contrary, thought she represented "an academic and emotional risk." To bolster his opinion, he pointed out that persons who have interrupted their college careers are less likely to graduate than persons who have not—ignoring the fact that Myra Lee did complete her college education, and with a nearly perfect record—and that persons who have attempted suicide are more likely to commit suicide than persons who have not—ignoring the fact that Myra Lee never seriously attempted to commit suicide.

Almost six months after the trial, Justice Nadel rendered his decision. As we had expected, he ruled that New York Medical College could quite properly reject Myra Lee Glassman's application for admission because of the interruption in her college education and because of her suicide "attempts," as he phrased it, "even though the interruption in the academic career resulted from, and the attempts at suicide resulted in, admission to a mental hospital." He had reached that decision, he said, because he believed that the mental hygiene law, which prohibited discrimination solely because of hospitalization, should be narrowly construed. Under such reasoning, prospective employers could say with impunity, "We are turning you down not because you were hospitalized, but because you were sick."

Suppose the statute said "no discrimination because of race" and the college said, "We are turning you down not because you are Negro, but because you have black skin and curly hair." Or suppose the statute said "no discrimination because of sex" and the college said, "We are turning you down not because you are female, but because you might become pregnant while in school." Is there any doubt such actions would be illegal? Certainly not. Race and sex are obviously shorthand terms for prohibiting a broad range of discriminatory acts. Similarly, we had argued that "admitted to a hospital" was simply a shorthand way of saying "seriously mentally ill." But Justice Nadel rejected that argument, ruling, curiously, that "to accept plaintiff's interpretation of Section 70 (5) of the Mental Hygiene Law would result in discrimination against all applicants who had not been patients in a mental hospital."

Finally, without bothering to distinguish the uncontradicted evidence of record, Justice Nadel embraced the college's aggregate of factors argument: "The decision to reject plaintiff's application was based upon her entire record, which included her grades, recommendations, tests, and personal interviews."

We could have appealed the decision. Perhaps we would have won in the long run. But by the time the decision was announced, Myra had applied to and been accepted by a midwestern medical school considerably more prestigious than New York Medical College, so we did not.

Recognizing that Myra was an exceptionally gifted student, the midwestern school offered her a substantial fellowship to participate in an unusual joint program combining the study of medicine and chemistry. Medical school would be hard enough by itself, and the joint program would be even more difficult. But upon graduation Myra would receive degrees in both medicine and pharmacology, becoming one of the few people in the United States with that kind of specialized training. She accepted.

Myra has now successfully completed two years of the program, earning honors in most of her courses and superior grades in all the rest.

Part IV
Getting There

Who shall decide when doctors disagree?
—ALEXANDER POPE
Moral Essays, Epistle III

Each state has its own statutes governing involuntary hospitalization. Some states require a court hearing before a person can be
sent to a hospital against his will. Others, including New York,
do not require judicial proceedings, but permit involuntary hospitalization whenever one or two physicians are willing to say
"this man is mentally ill"—whatever that means.

Many states require at least an allegation (though often little
proof) that the prospective patient is dangerous to himself or
others. But a large and growing number of states, including New

York, authorize the involuntary hospitalization of absolutely harmless people for their own "welfare."

Although the statutes vary, the same constitutional issues arise in almost every commitment proceeding. Some of those issues form the basis for the next two chapters.

11 / No Opinion

Catherine Henley was born in 1932 and graduated in 1953 from Wellesley College. Ten years later she was certified as a registered nurse, and shortly thereafter she married a man named Jonathan who was both ten years younger and a good deal less mature than she. By 1969, the marriage had become a very unhappy one, despite three children. Employed only occasionally, Jonathan was content to live on his wife's earnings and whatever pleasure he could take from constantly reminding her that she was "getting old." He disappeared for days at a time, sometimes weeks, and much of his time at home was spent lamenting his marriage to "an older woman."

Catherine Henley's failing marriage depressed her because, in spite of everything, she still loved Jonathan. Then, in the middle of June, 1969, Jonathan disappeared again, and on June 20, desperate for help, Mrs. Henley called a baby-sitter and took a taxi to the Mental Hygiene Clinic of Beth Israel Hospital, in the southeast quarter of Manhattan. There she asked to see a psychiatrist about her marital problems and deepening depression. She was told to come back the next morning.

On June 21, after locating another baby-sitter, she returned to Beth Israel and spoke with Dr. Arthur Ladli, who prescribed a tranquilizer and sleeping pills and suggested still another visit the following day. Mrs. Henley agreed to return. At ten the next morning, however, she telephoned Dr. Ladli to report that she was "tired," had been unable to find a baby-sitter, and "would make another appointment as soon as she could." Four days later, Dr. Ladli heard from her sister, Gwendolyn Rorach, that Catherine Henley had been neglecting the children—not feeding them or herself properly—and that she spent most of the day crying and walking aimlessly around her small apartment on East Fourth Street. Gwendolyn had gone to visit the Henleys earlier that morning, just as Jonathan, back home for a few hours, was leaving again. Gwendolyn thought her sister could use "a short rest" in a hospital, and Dr. Ladli agreed.

At noon the next day, June 27, Gwendolyn went to the Henley apartment, accompanied by two New York City police officers, Dr. Martin Karas, the Rorach family doctor, and George Fox, the Rorachs' lawyer. Mrs. Henley refused to let them in, but the police entered through a side window and took her to Bellevue Hospital's psychiatric division, where she was admitted on the strength of a "two-physician certificate" signed by Doctors Ladli and Karas. The certificate was a printed form, containing no facts. (Three weeks later, just before Catherine Henley's judicial hearing, Gwendolyn filled in the facts that supposedly had been the basis for the hospitalization.) Later that afternoon, Harmon Johnston, a Bellevue doctor, interviewed Mrs. Henley and found that "she was disheveled in her appearance, tearful, depressed, and restless." Three days later, Dr. Johnston interviewed her again and found that although she "felt she was railroaded to the hospital by the family" and was "suspicious and evasive," she "still was oriented [that is, she knew who she was, where she was, and what time it was], relevant, and coherent." Mrs. Henley insisted that Gwendolyn was "determined to put me in a state hospital and to separate me from my children and my husband," and Dr. Johnston could not persuade her otherwise.

On July 9, almost two weeks after her hospitalization, Jonathan Henley finally came to Bellevue, but only to tell Dr. Johnston that Mrs. Henley "needs hospital treatment; she is not able to function." Gwendolyn and her husband agreed with him.

Another week passed. According to Bellevue records, Catherine Henley spent most of her time "alone in a corner reading a book." Then, on July 15, she finally appeared in court for the judicial review of her hospitalization she had requested many days earlier. She was represented by Robert M. Hardy, an attorney employed by the Mental Health Information Service, an agency created by statute to assist mental patients in securing their rights. Also in the courtroom were Gwendolyn Rorach, Jonathan, Mrs. Henley's mother, and George Fox, the Rorachs' lawyer, all of whom opposed her discharge.

The hearing was brief. The first witness was Dr. Johnston, the Bellevue doctor, who testified for two and a half minutes. He reviewed the circumstances of Catherine Henley's admission to Bellevue and described her behavior on the ward. Before Johnston could recommend whether or not she should be hospitalized, Judge Abraham Gellinoff interrupted—"I don't think you have to go any further, Doctor"—and asked to hear from Dr. Martin Karas, one of the signers of the two-physician certificate

(Dr. Ladli, the other, did not testify). The interruption from the bench upset Robert Hardy's plans. He had wanted to cross-examine Dr. Johnston closely to find out whether outpatient treatment would not in fact have been more sensible for Catherine Henley than confinement. With Dr. Karas already on the stand and ready to talk, Hardy quickly asked Judge Gellinoff if he would have an opportunity later in the hearing "to ask some questions of Dr. Johnston." "Surely," said the judge.

Dr. Karas's testimony was equally brief. He had seen Mrs. Henley only once, on the day of her admission to Bellevue, and had no idea whether she had improved or deteriorated during her three weeks there, so he spoke only about the events preceding hospitalization. He had learned from Gwendolyn Rorach that there was "possible neglect of the children." He had arrived at the Henley apartment and found Mrs. Henley, "shaking, with her arms crossed." She had appeared "very angry, very anxious, very, very depressed, very concerned about her children—where they were in the room." She had "felt that her sister was trying to get the children from her." Karas, like Johnston, made no recommendation concerning hospitalization.

The next and final witness was Catherine Henley. Her testimony was articulate and to the point:

I had been under considerable stress. I have three young children, and my husband had recently left his job, and I was worried about that, and I noticed that I was getting overtired and a little distraught, so I went to Beth Israel to the emergency room and saw a doctor. He said I had to see him before I could see the psychiatrist, and he said to come to the Mental Hygiene Clinic the next morning, so I did and saw Dr. Ladli, and he gave me a prescription for a tranquilizer and sleeping pills. I was too tired to get there to keep the appointment the next morning, with three children, so I called and said I would make another appointment as soon as I could. I was handling the situation, and I do not believe hospitalization was necessary. I wasn't getting more tired; I was getting less tired. I was taking care of the children.

At that, Judge Gellinoff asked, "Do you think you are the real judge as to whether you need hospitalization?" Without waiting for an answer, he turned to the relatives. "What does the family propose to do? Where would they like to have her treated?"

In a few minutes it was over. Catherine Henley was committed for six months to the New York Hospital, Westchester Division, as her family had suggested. Hardy was given no opportunity to cross-examine Doctors Johnston and Karas, or even to raise the question of outpatient care.

A few days later, Hardy called my office and asked me to represent Mrs. Henley on appeal. He was angry that he had not been allowed to cross-examine the doctors. For this he partly blamed himself. But he was even more disturbed that she had been sent away for six months. As an MHIS lawyer with offices at Bellevue, he had seen and represented scores of patients; to him, it seemed clear that Catherine Henley's depression could have been treated adequately on an outpatient basis, and that hospitalization would only increase her depression. Gwendolyn Rorach had admitted to Hardy that she was pushing for hospitalization rather than outpatient treatment primarily because she wanted to separate Catherine Henley from her husband, who she thought was the cause of most of her sister's difficulties. George Fox, the family lawyer, told me later that the Rorachs despised Jonathan and hoped that the separation would enable Catherine to get over her futile and self-destructive love for him.

I told Hardy I would be happy to represent her. Since she had not yet been transferred to New York Hospital, I went immediately to Bellevue to meet her. She was on Ward NO-6, a treatment ward. She was tall, thin, and agitated. She clutched a worn paperback and talked intelligently of her eagerness to be discharged, expressing gratitude for my help. She was particularly upset because that morning Jonathan had come to tell her what she already suspected—that he did not love her, and adding, as he left, that he was filing for divorce.

The first step in our case was to demand a jury trial to review Judge Gellinoff's decision. The demand was filed on July 24. On the thirty-first, Judge Francis J. Bloustein ordered the court clerk to impanel a jury. However, because of the summer slowdown in the courts, the trial would not be scheduled before September 5. This meant that Mrs. Henley would be held in Bellevue for another month. And she would be held without treatment. As soon as she had demanded jury review, she was transferred from NO-6 to a nontreatment ward—in other words, a holding pen. The justification: "We can't treat patients who are demanding to get out."At that I exploded, pointing out that Bellevue had been treating Catherine Henley for a month, despite her repeated requests for release. When I threatened to sue, calling the transfer a punishment for exercising a constitutionally protected right, the Bellevue administration caved in and returned her to NO-6.

We had a good case, I thought. Several psychiatrists had agreed to testify before the jury that Catherine Henley did not need hospitalization, that outpatient treatment would suffice, indeed, would be better for her than the drab and depressing atmosphere of a mental hospital. On the day before the jury trial, after holding her for ten weeks, Bellevue suddenly decided that she did not need long-term hospitalization and discharged her. The reason for her discharge was obvious. Although every patient has a theoretical right to a jury trial, in New York there are never more than four or five a year; for most psychiatrists, a jury trial is such a nettlesome and time-consuming affair that the mere demand for one is usually enough to effect the patient's release.

Catherine Henley no longer had to worry about being sent to a state hospital. But the consequences of Judge Gellinoff's decision could plague her for the rest of her life. For one thing, armed with his decision, Gwendolyn Rorach had gone to family court and, with Jonathan's agreement, had obtained legal custody of the Henley children. In order to erase the stigma of mental illness, we appealed Judge Gellinoff's decision to a higher court, the Appellate Division, First Department. There was no way now to review the facts—a jury would have done that if Mrs. Henley had not been discharged—but we could still ask the appellate division to review the law, and to reverse Judge Gellinoff's decision because of an error of law.

Involved here was a simple but extraordinarily important legal point—the doctrine of less drastic alternatives. In countless decisions, the United States Supreme Court has ruled that "even though the governmental purpose be legitimate and substantial, that purpose cannot be pursued by means that broadly stifle fundamental personal liberties when the end can be more narrowly achieved. The breadth of legislative abridgement must be viewed in the light of less drastic means for achieving the same basic purpose." In other words, when there is more than one solution to a problem, the state must choose the one that least constricts individual rights. The less-drastic-alternatives doctrine is usually applied in cases where the state unnecessarily curtails freedom of speech, but, since it protects any fundamental personal liberty, the doctrine has also been applied to protect freedom of travel, the right to a passport, and a married couple's right to practice birth control.

In 1966, the federal appellate court for the District of Columbia, one of the country's most respected courts, ruled that the doctrine was applicable in "proceedings involving the care and treatment of the mentally ill." Specifically, before ordering full-time hospitalization, it was the "obligation of the state to bear the burden of exploration of possible alternatives." That decision, however, was not binding in New York. The Supreme Court had never had occasion to consider whether the doctrine applied in mental commitment cases, though it had recently criticized a juvenile court's failure to explore alternatives other than commitment. I saw close parallels between juvenile proceedings and psychiatric proceedings. Both involved deprivation of liberty; both were civil rather than criminal; in both, the ostensible purpose was treatment, not punishment; both created stigma; both involved aberrant behavior.

The appeal was argued in early February, 1970. I conceded that Catherine Henley had been depressed, even severely depressed, but I challenged Judge Gellinoff's assumption that a finding of depression, standing alone, justified long-term commitment to a state hospital. Doctors Johnston and Karas, the only doctors who testified, had not recommended such an extreme remedy. And no one had even considered less drastic alternatives, much less rejected them. Catherine Henley was an intelligent woman, a college graduate and a nurse. She had recognized her need for help and had, on her own initiative, made two trips to a psychiatric clinic to get it. Clearly, she was an excellent candidate for outpatient treatment. At least it had been worth a try; if she had failed to keep her clinic appointments, she could have been rehospitalized.

The five judges seemed miffed that such a troublesome constitutional issue had been laid in their laps. "But, Mr. Ennis, there is no indication in the record that outpatient treatment would, in fact, have worked."

"That's exactly the point, Your Honor. Because no one even considered alternatives, we can't tell from the record whether or not they would have worked. But Judge Gellinoff resolved that ambiguity against Catherine Henley. If the doctrine of less drastic alternatives means anything, it means that an individual cannot be deprived of his liberty, even for humane reasons, until after the court is convinced, on the basis of testimony, that no less drastic alternative will suffice. Here, there was no such testimony. The state failed to meet its burden of proof and the judgment committing Catherine Henley to a state hospital was therefore erroneous."

The judges were more irritated than impressed; nor were they eager to think deeply. We waited for a month, and then the decision came: "It is unanimously ordered and adjudged that the judgment so appealed from be and the same is hereby, in all things, affirmed." Nothing more. No opinion, no explanation of their decision, no guidelines for the future.

On April 8, 1970, I asked the appellate division's permission to appeal its decision to the Court of Appeals, the highest court in New York State. As a basis for the appeal, I argued that the applicability of the doctrine of less drastic alternatives to mental commitment proceedings was an issue of extraordinary and daily importance in the administration of New York's mental hygiene law. The issue was important not only to Catherine Henley, but also to thousands of persons hospitalized in New York each year. A month later, on May 12, the appellate division handed down a one-sentence order denying permission to appeal.

The next step was to ask the Court of Appeals itself for leave to appeal. In my briefs, I stressed the state-wide importance of the issue and all but begged the court to write an opinion. I was convinced that if the judges would only set hand to paper, would only think about the issue, we could not lose. On July 2, 1970, I received a telegram from the clerk of the Court of Appeals. It said, in full: MOTION FOR LEAVE TO APPEAL DENIED.

The Court of Appeals did not want to decide the case. And the appellate divsion, though it had been forced to decide, had done so without writing a word about whether the doctrine of less drastic alternatives applied to mental commitment cases. The judiciary's reluctance to get involved was not surprising. Courts do not like to grapple with new issues. I and others will continue to raise the issue of less drastic alternatives in new cases, and the courts no doubt will continue to ignore it until one day, convinced at last that the issue will not go away, some judge will be forced to sit down and think about what we have been saying. So it is in the practice of civil rights law. The occasional victory, however visible, is only the tip of the test-case iceberg. For every case decided by a court, hundreds are ignored.

Soon after her release from Bellevue, Catherine Henley found a job. A few weeks later she was recommitted—I do not know the circumstances. Once again, the Mental Health Information Service tried to get her out, and once again her family opposed. This time, however, the MHIS was successful and she was discharged. One week later, Catherine Henley threw herself in front of a subway train and died.

12 / Free the Bellevue Five Hundred

Bellevue Hospital's psychiatric division has only 500 beds, yet the patient turnover is so high that each year 10,000 to 15,000 persons are confined against their will within its walls, making Bellevue one of the busiest mental hospitals in the nation.

Bellevue serves as a social dumping ground for New York City's alcoholics, addicts, and Bowery bums. It takes in runaway teen-agers and college students on "bad trips," old people who can no longer walk or feed themselves, troublemakers, demonstrators, black men, white men, Chinese. It accepts the very depressed and the hyperactive and everything in between. It takes these people and sorts them out, sending most back to their park benches or welfare hotels, and a few on to state mental hospitals.

Most of my clients have spent time in Bellevue, and I have visited there often enough to be able to agree when they say it is not a pleasant place. Bellevue is too busy to treat patients as individuals. They must be quickly categorized and shunted on toward whatever disposition has been devised for persons in their category. If a patient has been brought to Bellevue from the Lower East Side of Manhattan, he will be shipped to Central Islip State Hospital, fifty miles east on Long Island. Patients from the Upper West Side of Manhattan will be sent to Rockland State Hospital, twenty miles north of the city—even those whose families happen to live near Central Islip.

At set times throughout the day, the patients in each ward form sullen lines and shuffle to the nursing cart, where each receives his paper cup of Thorazine. Most of the patients wear the same loose-fitting garb: blue pajama pants and top and white cloth slippers, each with "Bellevue" stenciled on it.

Nearly all the patients in Bellevue have problems that could be handled adequately in the community, or in some place other than a mental hospital. Very few need strictly psychiatric treatment. But it is easier to put people in Bellevue than to devise more personalized and less degrading solutions to their problems. Instead of building community mental health centers and decent nursing homes, we just add another wing to Bellevue so that additional persons can bear the label "mental patient."

If it were more difficult to put people in Bellevue, society would be forced to provide other solutions that would be better for them and, ironically, cheaper for us—the per-patient cost at Bellevue is nearly $100 a day. But it is not difficult to put people in Bellevue; it is astonishingly easy

This chapter is about a test case brought to restrict the kinds and numbers of persons who can be committed against their will to Bellevue and places like it. It was one of the first cases I brought, and clearly the most important. In asking that mental hospitals be made places of *last* resort, it called for a reversal of our mental health priorities. Today, three years after the case was filed, I have returned, by a rather circuitous route, to the same court where I started, still awaiting a favorable decision. So far, my clients and I have been defeated by the judicial process.

The cases described earlier were also test cases, brought not to enforce the law but to change it. They too were delayed and shaped and hindered by the judicial process; but the emphasis in those chapters was on the patients themselves and on the law, rather than on the process. It is important, however, not to slight the judicial process, because it often has more impact on the final outcome of a case than the facts or the law.

Everyone knows that the judicial process is slow. Perhaps less well known are the detrimental effects of delay on test cases in particular. Many drag on so long that the plaintiffs eventually give up hope and abandon their lawsuits. A man who has been denied a hack license because he was once a mental patient cannot afford to wait three years for a court to say that he should have been given the license. To support his family, he has to take the first available job, or move to another state where his past is less likely to be known. Many of the cases described here have not been finally resolved, and may not be for several years. If the older plaintiffs die before then, they will have gained nothing, not even the satisfaction of having changed the law so that others will not suffer what they did. I and other lawyers will have to start again, raising the same issues with new and younger plaintiffs.

This chapter, like the others, is about real people—Michael Fhagen and Mary Summers—but, unlike the others, the emphasis is on the judicial process. For that reason, it is more technical in its step-by-step description of the painstaking way an issue is finally brought before the higher courts for decision. The process is not unlike a war. Dozens of skirmishes must be won before the main battle is joined. It must first be proved that the court has jurisdiction, that the plaintiff has standing to raise the issue, that the defendant cannot claim any special defense such as sovereign immunity or official immunity, and so on.

These points may not seem central to the larger issues. Yet they embody the frustrations, the side issues, and the delays that are inherent in the judicial machinery, and explain why—even when lawyers for both sides are trying to speed a case along—the process takes years. The process therefore has the effect of discouraging test-case litigation and works to the advantage of the state, which is almost always in favor of the status quo.

The Civil Liberties Union does not charge fees. If I had been in private practice, the case described here would have cost the clients at least $10,000 to $15,000. Mental patients cannot pay such fees. And lawyers in private practice cannot afford to absorb that kind of loss. Thus, only a handful of lawyers, primarily those working for the Civil Liberties Union and similar organizations, are in a position to bring constitutional test-case litigation. This means, in turn, that most state policies and practices are effectively insulated from review. For the most part, mental hospitals, prisons, school boards, and welfare departments, to name a few, can do pretty much as they please without fear of a lawsuit. The occasional test case is just a drop in the bucket.

Even with the rare test case that is eventually won, the challenged practices, in violation of the constitutional rights of hundreds or thousands of persons, will probably have been continued during the intervening years. This chapter, for example, describes a challenge to the involuntary hospitalization provisions of the New York mental hygiene law. That law may ultimately be held unconstitutional, but in the meantime thousands of people will have been involuntarily hospitalized under it while the challenge was pending. For them, justice delayed will be justice denied.

If what I say about the judicial process is somewhat dry, that is precisely the point. For the most part, test-case litigation is dull, tedious work, requiring not brilliance, but endless hours of research and laborious attention to detail. If the system works, it works slowly and at great cost. This chapter, then, is more about the system than about Michael Fhagen and Mary Summers.

I first met Michael Fhagen in May of 1969, while he was a patient at Bellevue. Fhagen was one of the first mental patients I had ever seen, and he scared me. He scared everyone. He was not big, but he looked tough. Two of his front teeth were missing, and when he talked his otherwise boyish face took on a sinister edge. Moreover, he was aggressively loud and intense. I think it was the intensity that scared me, his habit of holding his face only inches away from whomever he was talking to, as if he did not recognize private space. It was impossible to avoid the urgency in his eyes. Everything was important. The slightest detail of the hospital routine and of the circumstances of his hospitalization had to be described precisely, exactly. As I talked, he wrote feverishly in a well-worn stenographer's notebook, transcribing word for word.

Later, I would learn that his peculiar intensity, which made him seem so threatening to others, was caused not by madness, but by a severe diabetic condition that occasionally flared out of control. It was usually during one of those flare-ups that Fhagen would find himself a patient in a mental hospital. Now he was hospitalized again, for the fourth time in seven years.

On Friday, April 28, 1969, Michael Fhagen had gone to the outpatient clinic of New York Hospital in upper Manhattan to pick up his regular two-week supply of insulin. On his way, he had been caught in a traffic jam, which prevented him from reaching the hospital until 5:50, ten minutes before closing time.

The employees in the medication office, eager to leave for the weekend, refused to fill his prescription. To a diabetic, insulin is life itself, and Fhagen was out of insulin. Without a new supply, he knew he could not survive the night, so he climbed the stairs to the diabetic clinic and asked a nurse what to do. She told him to go to the emergency room, explain the problem, and ask the doctor on duty to give him a one-day supply. By then, Fhagen was worried that without insulin he would soon go into shock, as he had many times before. Hurrying to the emergency room, he found several people waiting ahead of him. The doctors and nurses, apparently busy with other emergencies, paid no attention to him. After nearly an hour, Fhagen left and walked around the block to get some fresh air. When he returned, he again asked for help and again received no response. Now he was furious. He saw several young interns standing and chatting at the rear of the emergency room. His complaint that he was going into diabetic shock brought no response. Desperate, he pulled a window scraper out of his rear pocket (he was employed as a part-time painter) and began to bang it on the metal doorframe.

The interns responded by calling the police. Soon two officers arrived, searched Fhagen for narcotics, and took him to Bellevue, telling the admissions office there that Fhagen had gone to "N.Y. Hospital for medication for his diabetes, became very hostile, and threatened doctors with a razor blade." He was admitted as an emergency patient under section 78 of the New York mental hygiene law. The Bellevue records indicate that Fhagen was in diabetic shock. Immediately upon admission, he was put on 36 units of NPH, a diabetic medication. When he failed to respond, the dosage was increased to 70 units daily.

On May 21, I filed a petition in the state supreme court for a writ of habeas corpus, challenging the constitutionality of the statutes under which Fhagen had been hospitalized, together with a fifty-three-page brief crammed with cases and authorities supporting our position. The case was set for hearing on May 27 in the Bellevue courtroom. But when the judge discovered it was going to be a test case, he adjourned the hearing until June 3, over my objection. On the third, a different judge gave the hospital a second adjournment, this time for two weeks.

In protesting the additional delay, I pointed out that Fhagen had already been confined for over five weeks without any judicial hearing. I stressed that in our view this constituted an illegal confinement. The judge's reply was quick, if not very persuasive. "You think you're pretty smart, don't you?" he said, and ordered me to sit down. He would not even require the hospital to answer or deny the allegations of the habeas corpus petition, which it is supposed to do within three days, or to furnish us with an answering brief demonstrating in what respects, if any, the hospital took issue with the legal arguments raised in our brief. In other words, at the next hearing, the hospital's lawyers would arrive in court knowing everything we would try to prove; we would arrive cold, knowing nothing at all about the hospital's position.

Discouraged by the hostility of two successive state court judges, Fhagen and I decided to try other ways to get him out of the hospital. By now his diabetic condition had stabilized to the point that we were able to wangle a pass permitting him one day of freedom from Bellevue. He went immediately to New York Hospital and was examined by two psychiatrists, who gave him a letter agreeing to accept him as an outpatient.

Fhagen then returned to Bellevue, and I arranged to meet with Dr. Yorihiko Kumasaka, the psychiatrist on his ward. I asked Kumasaka if he considered Fhagen suitable for outpatient treatment. "No," he replied. "He's too sick for that. He will have to be sent to a state hospital for at least six months." I told Kumasaka about the pass and the letter. "Impossible," he said. "Mr. Fhagen could not have left Bellevue without my knowledge or permission." I told Kumasaka that unless he wanted to look foolish at Fhagen's judicial hearing, he had better check with the ward nurse. When she showed him the letter, he agreed to discharge Fhagen.

On June 12, Fhagen left Bellevue without having appeared in court, and his habeas corpus proceeding was dismissed as moot. Fhagen, however, did not want to stop there. He had been hospitalized four times under the New York statutes and was afraid it would happen again. He asked me to bring a lawsuit seeking to have the court declare those statutes unconstitutional.

Because of our chilly reception in state court, I decided to bring the case in federal court. This I did on July 22, 1969. The defendants, the director of Bellevue and the state commissioner of mental hygiene, were supposed to answer the complaint within twenty days, either admitting or denying its allegations. As usual, however, they requested an extension. I agreed to three months, partly because if I had refused, the court would no doubt have granted a month or two anyway, and partly because I wanted the case decided by Judge Edward Weinfeld, an exceptionally competent man, who would be presiding in the "motion part" three months from then.

Normally, federal cases are decided by a single judge, but a federal statute forbids a federal judge, acting alone, from enjoining or prohibiting the enforcement of a state statute. We were seeking to enjoin the enforcement of two state statutes—sections 72 and 78 of the mental hygiene law—which together accounted for about 95 per cent of all involuntary hospitalizations in New York. Thus it was necessary to request a special three-judge federal court. I waited until Judge Weinfeld was sitting and then, on October 16, 1969, asked him to convene a three-judge court, of which he would be a member.

It is one thing to request a three-judge court and another to get one. Before one judge will impose on two of his already overworked colleagues, he must be persuaded that the constitutional arguments raised by the plaintiff are, at least, substantial. In fact, he must think that the plaintiff has a good chance of winning. In order to convince Judge Weinfeld that our arguments were substantial, I submitted a memorandum of law that pointed out several defects in the New York commitment statutes.

The main defect was that a person could be hospitalized against his will under sections 72 and 78 without any opportunity, prior to hospitalization, to appear before a judge to tell his side of the story. Fhagen had initially been hospitalized under section 78, which authorized hospitals to confine persons for thirty days whenever they were "alleged to be in need of immediate observation, care or treatment for mental illness." The law was silent about who could make such an allegation. In practice, it could be made, and usually was, by a layman. It did not have to be confirmed by a doctor or approved by a judge. Nor did the allegation have to be made in writing or under oath. A phone call from a neighbor would do.

After the thirty days, a person could be held against his will for another sixty days if two physicians—they need not be psychiatrists—signed a piece of paper saying that, in their opinion, he was mentally ill. That was what had happened to Fhagen.

Persons confined under section 78 did not have the right, even after hospitalization, to ask a court to examine the propriety of their hospitalization. For that, they had to wait for conversion to section 72 status—that is, until after two doctors had certified that they were mentally ill. Only then did they have the right to request a judicial hearing. And if they did not make such a request in writing, they could be held for the rest of their lives without ever appearing before a judge.

Fhagen had been hospitalized before. He knew through experience what his rights were. Most mental patients are ignorant of their right to request judicial review. Or they are so drugged by the tranquilizers the hospitals routinely administer, or so dazed and confused from shock therapy, or so cowed by their doctors, that they are unable, or afraid, to assert themselves. In one year, for example, Bellevue admitted 15,000 involuntary patients, of whom only 531 requested judicial review. In other words, the right to judicial review was little more than a theoretical right, a right that existed only on paper. If, for whatever reason, the patient did not file a written request for a court hearing or for a lawyer, he was deemed by his inaction to have waived, or given up, those rights.

In this regard, the legal protections for mental patients were years behind the protections afforded other classes of people who might be locked up. The law was clear with respect to alleged criminals, and alleged narcotics addicts, and alleged juvenile delinquents: they were not deemed to have waived their rights to a lawyer or to a court hearing unless they had affirmatively said they did not want a lawyer or a hearing. Furthermore, the courts would not accept even an affirmative waiver unless convinced that it had been made "knowingly and intelligently." It was inconceivable to me that a person alleged to be under mental disability could knowingly and intelligently waive his right to a lawyer or a hearing by mere inaction. That could not be the law.

On October 22, 1969, instead of filing an answer, Bellevue and the Department of Mental Hygiene filed a memorandum of law and a motion to dismiss the complaint. They contended that because Fhagen had been discharged, the action was moot and he lacked standing to challenge the commitment statutes, that the defendants were immune from this kind of lawsuit, and that, in any event, the constitutional arguments we had raised were not substantial.

The next day, I filed a reply memorandum, which attempted to point out weaknesses in the defendants' arguments.

Our motion to convene a three-judge court and their motion to dismiss the complaint were argued before Judge Weinfeld on November 21, 1969. On December 4, he denied their motion, granted ours, and ruled that our constitutional arguments were indeed substantial.

Now I had to prepare a much more detailed brief for submission to the three-judge court. The brief was filed the day before Christmas. The defendants' answering brief was due on January 7, 1970, but they asked for a three-week extension, which the court granted. At the end of January, they asked for two more weeks, which were also granted.

On February 11, 1970, apparently convinced by the tone of Judge Weinfeld's opinion that the federal court was on the verge of striking down major portions of the mental hygiene law, defendant Alan Miller, the commissioner of mental hygiene, issued an administrative regulation that changed the hospitalization provisions in several respects. The maximum period of emergency hospitalization was reduced from thirty days to fifteen. Although still permitting the allegation of a layman to initiate the hospitalization process, the regulation required for the first time that prospective patients be examined by a doctor before admission. Also for the first time, emergency patients were granted the right to obtain judicial review of their hospitalization, and had to be given notice of this and other rights.

Two days later the defendants filed a rather hefty brief (fifty-three pages) claiming that the state laws governing involuntary hospitalization were constitutional. More important, however, they maintained that the three-judge court should abstain—that is, the federal court should not decide the case, but should send it back to the state courts. Their argument, in essence, was that the new regulation had modified the state statutes to such an extent as to make the law governing involuntary hospitalization unclear, and that the state courts were in a better position to decide exactly what the state law now was. It might be, they said, that the state courts would construe the statutes in a way that would answer many, or all, of the plaintiff's objections. For example, although the "emergency" statute did not expressly require an allegation that the prospective patient was dangerous, the state courts, said the defendants, might construe that statute to require an allegation of dangerousness, thus eliminating one of plaintiff Fhagen's objections.

I did not want the federal court to abstain. Our reception in state court had been so hostile—two state court judges had refused to rule on Fhagen's petition—that I saw no hope there. On February 25, 1970, in an effort to persuade the federal court to keep the case, I made a motion to add Mary Summers (see chapter eight) as a second plaintiff. I did this because I thought the federal court might be more sympathetic to her than to Fhagen, and thus more inclined to keep the case.

Mary Summers, it will be remembered, had been taken to Bellevue as an emergency patient because she had refused to move from one hotel room to another. Unlike Fhagen, she was not loud or aggressive. In fifty-eight years, she had never before been hospitalized. She stayed in her room reading her Bible and minding her own business. She had never threatened or injured anyone, and since she got a room with a private bath, she had lived in peace with her neighbors. I knew that Fhagen had not threatened doctors with a razor blade, but the Bellevue records said he had, and I was afraid the judges would be troubled by that allegation. Mary Summers, on the other hand, would elicit only sympathy. It was not surprising, therefore, that the defendants opposed her addition as a plaintiff.

On March 13, 1970, I filed a sixty-two-page reply brief pointing out the many reasons why the federal court should not abstain. The case law was clear, for example, that federal courts were the primary forum for vindication of federal constitutional rights, that "cases involving vital questions of civil rights are the least likely candidates for abstention," and that sending a case back to the state courts was particularly inappropriate "where the constitutional challenge is sufficiently substantial [as it was in our case] to require the convening of a three-judge court."

The case was argued on April 7 before Judge Weinfeld and Judges Irving R. Kaufman and Edmund L. Palmieri. Two weeks later, the three-judge court announced that it had decided to abstain. All three judges indicated doubts about the constitutionality of the state statutes. Their abstention was based solely on their belief that "state court construction could well eliminate or at least present in a radically different posture the federal constitutional questions presented."

I was disappointed. Had the federal court kept the case, it would probably have decided in our favor and struck down the mental hygiene law as unconstitutional. But I had learned a lot in the eleven months the case had been pending. I had a better idea of the arguments the defendants would use in supporting the mental hygiene law. And I had learned more about how the law worked in practice. For example, I had learned that whereas section 78 had been intended to apply only to emergency hospitalizations, it was, in fact, the standard means of hospitalization in almost 98 per cent of the cases in New York City. The New York State legislature had probably not meant to foster the mass hospitalization—about 80,000 people a year—that was then taking place under the state mental hygiene law. Moreover, I now realized that to satisfy the requirement that patients be given notice of their rights it was common practice for hospital officials to slip the printed notice into the patient's hospital record and consider him notified, even though the patient did not have access to his record. Armed with this knowledge, I was able to draft a much more detailed complaint, one that specified additional objections to the mental hygiene law and that was phrased in such a way as to blunt some of the expected defenses. Naming Fhagen and Mary Summers as co-plaintiffs, that complaint was filed in the state supreme court on June 22, 1970.

Defendant Miller, the commissioner of mental hygiene, filed his answer on July 15, and defendant Alexander Thomas, the director of Bellevue, answered on July 24. They admitted most of the factual allegations of the complaint but denied that the mental hygiene law was unconstitutional.

Three days later, I made a motion for summary judgment, pointing out that there was no real factual dispute (and thus no need for a trial), and that the case was therefore ready to be decided on the legal issues. I scheduled the motion to be argued on August 14, two weeks later, when Justice Francis J. Bloustein would be sitting in Special Term Part I, the "motion part."

Now things got busy. The lawyers for the defendants planned to begin their vacations on August 14, the last day of Judge Bloustein's term. Predictably, they requested a one-month adjourn-ment. An examination of the list of judges who would follow Bloustein in Part I and a reading of some of their opinions con-vinced me that we would not have a fighting chance with anyone other than Judge Bloustein for another four or five months. So I made a deal. Rather than wait those four or five months in or-der to present oral argument, I offered to submit the case to Judge Bloustein on the fourteenth without oral argument. That way, the lawyers for the defendants would not have to be present in court. I would appear, tell the clerk in Special Term Part I that the case was submitted, and that would be it. The defend-ants agreed to this shortcut.

Since there would be no oral argument, it was important that the briefs be quite complete. On the twenty-ninth, two days after I had made the motion for summary judgment, I filed a seventy-two-page brief. On August 11, the defendants filed a motion re-questing summary judgment in their favor. On the twelfth, they filed a fifty-five-page brief. The next day, I filed a twenty-nine-page reply brief. On the fourteenth, I submitted all those papers to the clerk.

Almost four months later, on December 9, Judge Bloustein announced his decision. He ruled in our favor on a few minor points, but against us on most of the major ones. In retrospect, I probably was wrong to submit such an important case without oral argument. All the legal points had been made in the briefs, but clearly Judge Bloustein had not become emotionally involved in the issues. The main value of oral argument is to stress the hu-man dimensions, to remind the judge that the case is not about names, figures, and statistics, but about real people with real grievances. A good oral argument can spark a judge's sense of in-justice, of moral outrage; it can color his perceptions of the dry legal issues. That sense of outrage was missing from Judge Blou-stein's opinion.

Technically, the losing side cannot appeal from an adverse

opinion. It must wait until the judge signs another piece of paper, called an order, or a judgment. The order came down on January 28, 1971. Later that day I filed a notice of appeal.

The next step would be to "perfect" the appeal, a time-consuming and, in most cases, expensive process. All of the important papers filed in the court whose decision is being appealed must be collected, indexed, and printed in a document called an appendix. Several printed copies of the brief to the appellate court are also needed. Printing takes time and costs a lot of money. Printing the appeal papers in Edna Dalton Long's case, for example, cost my office about $1,500. But if the appellate court can be satisfied that the client is indigent, it may permit an appeal as a "poor person," which means the original papers can be filed with the appellate court, without the need for printing extra copies. In such circumstances, typewritten or xeroxed briefs are offered in place of printed briefs.

On February 11, I made a motion for permission to proceed as a poor person, supported by the affidavits of Michael Fhagen and Mary Summers that they were both on welfare and had no money. On March 4, the Appellate Division, First Department, which decides appeals from cases arising in Manhattan, granted that motion.

On March 15, I filed a judicial subpoena *duces tecum* and a certificate, which authorized the clerk of the lower court to transfer the original papers to the clerk of the appellate court. Two weeks later, I filed twenty-one xeroxed copies of a sixty-six-page brief. On April 20, the defendants filed a thirty-seven-page answering brief, and one week later I filed a nineteen-page reply brief.

The appeal was argued in the appellate division on May 5, 1971. I could tell immediately that the five judges on the court were not particularly sympathetic. I started my argument by pointing out that the state had just reduced the operating budget of the Department of Mental Hygiene by approximately $100 million. The cutback was so severe that even Commissioner Miller, one of the defendants, had publicly acknowledged that "many patients" would "not receive needed treatment, many would be poorly cared for," and "some would die." And the directors of five of the state mental hospitals had openly stated that because of the cutback "treatment would come to a grinding halt." The point, I said, was that the judges should be under no illusion about the quality of care in the state mental hospitals. They should face up to the fact that persons hospitalized under sections 78 and 72, allegedly for their own welfare, would be sent to institutions more closely resembling prisons than hospitals. At that point, one of the judges interrupted to ask, "Well, maybe they wouldn't get the treatment they should get, but what are we supposed to do about that? We can't just let all these dangerous people out on the streets."

I started to explain that even the defendants would admit that less than 5 per cent of the patients in their hospitals could be considered dangerous, and that we were challenging the constitutionality of sections 72 and 78 precisely because those sections authorized the involuntary hospitalization of absolutely harmless people. I hadn't finished that point, however, when a second judge interrupted to say that he didn't know what he, as a judge, could do to improve the lot of "these poor unfortunates." Before I could reply to his patronizing remark, a third judge added that he saw this as "a medical question, which we ought to leave to the doctors." And so it went. I was not surprised when, one week later, the appellate division unanimously affirmed Judge Bloustein's decision without an opinion.

On May 24, I filed a notice of appeal to the New York Court of Appeals, the highest court in the state. On the twenty-fifth, I asked the Court of Appeals, as I had earlier asked the appellate division, for permission to appeal as poor persons. At the same time, I also requested an expedited appeal, pointing out that for each year of delay literally thousands of people would be hospitalized under the statutes we were challenging.

On June 10, 1971, the Court of Appeals granted permission to appeal as poor persons but denied an expedited appeal. We would have to wait our turn on the appeal calendar, and since the Court of Appeals does not sit during the summer months, that meant waiting until fall.

On July 13, I filed a seventy-nine-page appellate brief and a thirty-three-page appendix which quoted and summarized the emergency hospitalization provisions for each of the fifty states and the District of Columbia. The purpose of the appendix was to let the seven judges of the court see for themselves the truth of my assertion that it was easier to have someone hospitalized against his will in New York than in any other state.

Three months later, on October 15, 1971, a Friday, the defendants filed a fifty-two-page answering brief. Oral argument was scheduled for the following Tuesday. That morning, I took the early bus to Albany, where the Court of Appeals sits, and filed the sixteen-page reply brief I had prepared over the weekend. The judges were courteous but gave no indication of how they felt about the case.

On January 6, 1972, the Court of Appeals unanimously affirmed the decisions of the lower courts upholding the constitutionality of the mental hygiene law. The opinion was about as short as it could be. We had presented five arguments, each supported by numerous court decisions from other states. Without discussing any of those decisions, the Court of Appeals dismissed our first two arguments in a page or two, and rejected the remaining arguments with a sentence: "We have examined the plaintiffs' other arguments and find them without substance."

Two weeks later, I filed a motion in federal court asking the three judges who had abstained twenty-one months earlier to resume consideration of the case. I pointed out that "the intervening proceedings in the state courts have shed little if any light on the issues before this court." The defendants, however, contended that since the state courts had now ruled upon their claims, Michael Fhagen and Mary Summers should not get a second chance in the federal district court. The three federal judges agreed, and dismissed the complaint.

I immediately sat down to draft a petition for a writ of certiorari, asking the United States Supreme Court to review the case. In all probability, the Supreme Court would decline to hear the case, leaving the legal issues unresolved. In that event, I would have to start again with new plaintiffs, a new complaint, and the prospect of additional years of delay. A federal court would someday rule on the constitutionality of the mental hygiene law, but even a favorable decision would come too late for Michael Fhagen and Mary Summers.

Part V
Impressions

The hidden stone finds the plough.
—ESTONIAN PROVERB

During the past three years, hundreds of patients and former patients have asked me for legal help. Often I could do nothing. Sometimes a letter or a telephone call was enough to get them out, or keep them out, of a mental hospital. Very few of those cases reached court, and many of those that did were either lost or, more frequently, won on such narrow grounds that the decisions did benefit anyone other than the person directly involved. A few of the cases described here changed the law. Those that follow did not. Many of them never reached court. They are worth remembering, nonetheless, because each gives us a clearer picture of the mental patient's world.

Anyone who lived in New York City between 1940 and 1957 will remember reading about George P. Metesky, known as "the Mad Bomber," who allegedly planted sixty bombs in an effort to gain revenge against the Consolidated Edison Company.

In 1931, while working for Con Edison, Metesky had been knocked down in a blast of hot air from a furnace in a Con Edison boiler room. He collapsed and vomited blood. Two days later he developed tuberculosis, which he attributed to the boiler-room incident. Con Edison refused to pay him anything and he was denied workmen's compensation.

No one was killed by the bombs Metesky allegedly set, but several people were injured. Metesky was arrested and indicted in both Kings and New York counties, and in March, 1957, he was found by a court to be competent to stand trial in New York County. In April, however, a different court found him to be incompetent to stand trial in Kings County, and he was committed to Matteawan.

During the next twelve years he tried several times to stand trial on the criminal charges, but each time the court found him still incompetent.

I do not know if he was guilty. I never asked, and he never told me. I do know that there was little evidence against him other than what he himself had supplied. Because of various United States Supreme Court decisions, much of that evidence could not have been used against him at a trial, and the state would have had a very hard time gaining a conviction.

This lack of evidence may be, at least in part, why a series of judges refused Metesky's repeated requests to stand trial. I could think of no other reason, because it was absolutely clear to me that he was competent to stand trial. Alert, intelligent, and articulate, Metesky knew much more than most defendants about the criminal process. Gene Ann Condon, who had handled his case without fee since 1966, had asked me to help. As a first step, we retained two psychiatrists, Jonathan Cohen and Ann Keill, who examined Metesky and reported that in their opinion he was quite competent to stand trial.

Despite these encouraging psychiatric opinions, we were convinced that we could not win on that factual issue before the same state court judges who had turned Metesky down so many times in the past. It seemed best to file a habeas corpus proceeding in federal court, one that raised legal issues. The case was argued before Judge Walter R. Mansfield on February 10, 1970.

On March 13, 1,000 persons (including, I was told, Judge Mansfield) were forced to evacuate the federal courthouse because of a bomb threat. On May 6, Judge Mansfield ruled against us.

Gene Ann Condon filed a notice of appeal and was ready to go on. But Metesky was not. Obviously discouraged by losing the habeas corpus proceeding, he wrote her that he had decided to stop taking the heart medication he needed to live, and would "let nature take its course."

Cleophus Charles was blind and black and a student at Cornell University. When, in 1969, several of his black brothers armed themselves with rifles and seized a campus building to protest racism at the university, Charles wanted to help. He certainly couldn't handle a gun, so he made a stack of sandwiches, established himself in the auditorium, and began round-the-clock discussions, with anyone who would listen, about the problems caused by racism at Cornell. School officials took him to the school clinic and, over his objection, gave him an injection to calm him down. The medication affected his sense of balance and, being blind, he lost his orientation, fell, and began to scream in outraged helplessness. The officials took him to a mental hospital, silencing his protest. It took a month, but we got him back in school.

I remember the hundreds of little ways in which patients were treated like children, or criminals, or worse. Frequently, for example, it was impossible to speak to a patient by telephone. On July 16, 1970, I decided to record a typical episode.

I called Grasslands Hospital to talk to a client who had been hospitalized for the second time in six months. When the ward nurse answered, I explained who I was and whom I was calling. My client, it turned out, was standing right by the telephone, but the ward nurse would not let me speak to her. "I'm sorry, patients cannot receive calls."

When I insisted, she switched the call to the head nurse. "I'm sorry, patients cannot receive calls."

Although I was not surprised—it happened all the time—I tried to sound amazed. "You mean to tell me that she can't even speak to her own lawyer?"

"No, not without the doctor's permission."

"Well, then, may I speak to the doctor?"

"No, he isn't here now."

I asked to be transferred to the director of the hospital. After some confusion, an unidentified woman answered, and I repeated the problem. "I would like to speak with my client, who is a patient," and so on.

She thought for a while—after all, this was so irregular!—and proposed that I call the head of the psychiatric division, Dr. Gails, for permission.

My call was again transferred, and I spoke with an evasive secretary.

"Dr. Gails is out for the day."

Once more I explained the problem and all the prior phone conversations, and she said she would look for a doctor.

No doctor. "Can I take your name and number and have someone call you? Because calls to patients must be approved by a doctor."

I told her that my client's judicial hearing was Monday, which it was, and that I needed to confer with her right away.

"Well, maybe Dr. Tessler can help you out."

I was transferred back to Ward 2N, where we had started.

"Bruce Menace?" the nurse queried.

"Not Menace—Ennis."

A long wait. At last, Dr. Amato took the phone and very efficiently took a message for my client, promising to have her call me immediately "from the patient phone."

Time elapsed: twenty-two minutes and forty-five seconds.

———

Edward Hunt received a B.A. in science and chemical engineering from New York University. He was an accomplished musician, and supported himself and his aging mother—they lived in an old frame house in New Jersey—by working sporadically as a clerk and by composing and selling music. But his real interest was mathematics.

By meticulous computation based on the life spans of Jared, Enoch, Methuselah, and Lamech, as revealed in the Bible— Genesis, chapter 5, starting with verse 6—Hunt had determined that the seven-year period (seven was a pivotal number) between 1962 and 1969—which corresponded to the 962 years of Jared and the 969 years of Methuselah—was to be the "Great Sabbath." Other facts were marshaled to support his theories. Thus, the Jewish people regained Israel on the fifth day of the sixth month of 1967, which corresponded to chapter 5, verse 6, and the always powerful number seven. The United States had fifty states, one for each of the fifty chapters of Genesis. And so on.

One day, when Hunt was in New York peacefully jotting down the number of persons who had used a particular subway turnstile on a particular day, a transit patrolman asked what he was doing. Hunt cheerfully handed him a four-page tract on his theories, and for his pains was immediately taken to Bellevue. From there he was transferred to Manhattan State and held for several months, until he demanded a jury trial.

Hunt had protested his hospitalization, pointing out that if he could not work to pay the rent on the house, he and his mother would be evicted. A Bellevue psychiatrist had told him that "a furnished room is good enough for you." They lost the house.

I remember a wizened little Czechoslovakian woman who claimed to be clairvoyant. Years ago she went to the police and offered to help solve a murder by using her psychic powers. They took her to Bellevue. From there she was sent to Manhattan State and then to Middletown, where she spent more than twenty years scrubbing floors and bathing incontinent patients. Every once in a while a doctor would come through the ward and ask if she still believed in her supernatural powers. She would say yes, and her commitment would continue. One day, it occurred to her that if she lied, she might be released. The next time a doctor asked if she still had her powers, she said no. A week later she was discharged.

Although her story seemed fantastic, I believed it because I learned it only indirectly, after much questioning. She was not at all upset by the apparent reason for her long confinement and did not even want to talk about it. She simply wanted my help in recovering some property that had been lost during her hospitalization.

Two months later, she returned to say she had received a "message" that her property would soon be recovered by the state police; she would no longer need my help.

One day in 1969, a shy, white-haired, red-faced old Irishman sat in my office and told me that he had just "escaped" from Pilgrim State Hospital. He had been held there, he said, for thirty-one years and was afraid he would be caught and taken back.

I checked with the hospital and found that he had indeed been there thirty-one years, though he had not escaped. Two years earlier, the hospital had converted him from involuntary to informal status. For two years he had been free to leave at any time, but no one had bothered to tell him.

Epilogue

The only freedom which deserves the name, is that of pursuing our own good in our own way, so long as we do not attempt to deprive others of theirs, or impede their efforts to obtain it. Each is the proper guardian of his own health, whether bodily, or mental and spiritual. Mankind are greater gainers by suffering each other to live as seems good to themselves, than by compelling each to live as seems good to the rest. —JOHN STUART MILL

It is worth repeating that the stories in this book are not unusual. Not at all. They were chosen not because they are particularly shocking, but because they are so typical of what it means to be a mental patient in the United States.

I could have reported stories it makes me sick, even now, to remember. Stories of disturbed ten-year-old boys beaten by attendants with baseball bats and threatened by nurses with castration if they did not behave; stories of the sexual exploitation, and sometimes murder, of confused and drugged patients; stories of such cruelty that they might not be believed. I did not include them because they are not what this book is about. Even if all the abuses of the mental hospital system could be eliminated, the system would still remain, and it is the system that must be changed.

When I came to the Civil Liberties Union to direct its Civil Liberties and Mental Illness Litigation Project, I knew there would be abuses of the system—I had been told that. I did not know the abuses were endemic to the system, that the system itself was a failure. It takes time to learn the facts. But they are there, if you are interested, and they are very dismal.

Society's ability to treat people with serious mental problems is no greater today than it was fifteen years ago. In 1955, for example, 78 per cent of all patients in New York State mental hospitals had been hospitalized for longer than two years. In 1970, the figure was 76 per cent. Not much of an improvement.

It is true that during the last decade the period of hospitalization in those hospitals declined from an average of several months to sixty days. But that is not so much due to improvements in treatment methods as it is to the fact that we are hospitalizing more and more people who are only mildly disturbed, people who should not be hospitalized at all. They are kept for a day or two and then discharged, which lowers the average hospital stay.

It follows that most mental hospitals in effect are two separate institutions—the low-turnover back wards for old, chronic, or seriously disturbed patients, and the high-turnover admissions wards for the young, the acutely ill, and the mildly disturbed.

The real tragedy of the mental hospital system is that few of the patients in the back wards get better, and many of the patients in the front wards get worse. It is now beyond dispute— even among psychiatrists—that prolonged hospitalization is, in itself, antitherapeutic. The patient who has successfully adapted to the structured, authoritarian world of the mental hospital would find it difficult to adapt again to the real world, and that difficulty decreases his chances of ever being discharged. Mental hospitals train people to be dependent, irresponsible, second-class citizens.

Fiorello LaGuardia, when he was mayor of New York City, said, "The worst home is better than the best mental hospital." He was right. Dozens of studies confirm that persons who are treated (or just ignored) *in their communities* improve faster and stay well longer than those who are treated in mental hospitals. In similar studies conducted in New York City and in Denver, persons who had already been screened and approved for hospital admission were randomly assigned to two groups. The first group was hospitalized; the second was sent back to the community for outpatient treatment. After two years, it was clear that the out-patient group was doing much better than the inpatient group— and was costing the state only half as much. In short, it makes no sense to put people in mental hospitals. It is bad for them and expensive for us.

There are other problems with the system. For one thing, we are no closer today to an understanding of mental illness than we were thirty years ago. The battles that raged then—battles over definition, cause, and cure—still rage today. If anything, they rage more intensely, for the spotlight has at last been turned on the miserable places society has spawned to rid itself of this trouble-some problem. Some psychiatrists see genetics as the root cause of mental illness, others blame it on chemical or hormonal im-balances, and still others point to early childhood traumas. A few, with much reason, deny the existence of such a thing as mental illness. They say it is either a physiological illness or a learned pattern of maladaptive behavior.

This uncertainty about causes carries over into *identification*. Psychiatrists and psychologists simply cannot agree among them-selves which persons are and which are not mentally ill. "Mental illness" is such an ambiguous term that it can, and does, mean whatever the examiner wants it to mean. The other terms used in psychiatry—schizophrenia, manic-depressive psychosis, paranoia, inappropriate affect, and so on—are equally vague and susceptible to abuse. But psychiatrists and judges who use such flexible terms to label people mad should not be singled out for blame. They are themselves products of a society that has always taken a rather narrow view of "normal" behavior.

Most of us fear what is different. That is understandable. We also fear criminals. But consider the difference between criminal laws and mental hygiene laws. We do not tolerate vagueness in the criminal law. We do not incarcerate people because they are criminal types, whatever that means, but because they have committed specific illegal acts—stealing a car, selling heroin, assaulting someone.

On the other hand, in a mental commitment case, the prospective patient is not charged with committing any specific act capable of proof or disproof. He is charged with being mentally ill or dangerous. If he is hospitalized, it is usually not because of something he has done, but because of a status attributed to him by a psychiatrist. His liberty is therefore dependent upon the personal values and biases of the particular psychiatrist who examines him.

Some psychiatrists believe that all hippies are mentally ill. Others disagree. Some psychiatrists believe that a person is "dangerous to himself" if he eats too much (or too little), or smokes cigarettes. Others limit the label to persons who have attempted suicide in the more conventional manner—slashing a wrist, or jumping from a window. British psychiatrists, when shown films of potential patients, tend to label mentally ill those who are unusually active or aggressive. American psychiatrists, viewing the same films, tend to pick out those who are unusually withdrawn and nonaggressive.

Obviously, the cultural background of the examiner weighs heavily in his evaluation of a prospective patient. Our mental hospitals are filled with foreign doctors, raised and trained—often inadequately—in cultures quite different from our own. Forty per cent of the doctors in New York state mental hospitals are not licensed to engage in the private practice of medicine in New York. Yet we consider these doctors, who in private practice could not lawfully treat patients, good enough for public hospital patients.

The examination administered by the Educational Council for Foreign Medical Graduates requires at least a minimum knowledge of English and medicine. But many public mental hospitals are staffed by doctors who cannot pass even that test, much less meet state licensing requirements. Although nationwide figures are not available, we know that the public mental hospitals of eleven states now employ almost 500 doctors who have not passed the Foreign Medical Graduates Examination.

Moreover, the better-trained and more competent doctors rise rapidly to administrative positions, where they rarely see patients. Thus, while unlicensed doctors may constitute only a minority of a hospital's staff, they are frequently the only doctors at the ward level. If a ward doctor cannot even understand English, it will be little comfort to his patients that the hospital director is a diplomate of the American Board of Psychiatry and Neurology.

The communication problems are formidable, especially between lower-class or black "street people" and their doctors— whether they be foreign-born or white middle-class Americans. A Bellevue doctor told me he once heard a Bellevue psychiatrist, who was Japanese, ask a prospective patient, "What does mean, a stitch in time gathers no moss?" The patient, who was dumbfounded by the question, was eventually committed. But beyond the language difficulty is a more fundamental problem. There are different norms even within our own culture. Behavior and language that would be quite normal in Harlem may seem seriously abnormal to a psychiatrist who lives in Scarsdale. Accepted behavior on a college campus—smoking marijuana, for example— might suggest to a sixty-five-year-old psychiatrist the presence of a serious underlying mental disorder.

The standards for involuntary hospitalization are terribly ambiguous. Each psychiatrist resolves that ambiguity in his own way, based on his own values and his preference for a safe society or a free society. The mental hospital system is governed not by laws, but by men who make their own laws.

In many states, a person can be hospitalized against his will whenever two physicians—they do not have to be psychiatrists—certify that in their opinion he is mentally ill. There is no standard against which to measure the accuracy of that opinion. In effect, you are mentally ill if two doctors—an obstetrician and a cardiologist, for instance—say you are. And once they say you are mentally ill, whatever that may mean to them, the entire power of the state can be called forth to enforce their private opinion.

Suppose the statute said a person could be hospitalized against his will whenever two lawyers or two mechanics or two school-teachers said that in their opinion he was mentally ill. Society would not tolerate such a statute. Yet the analogy is not so far-fetched. Doctors may couch their judgments in medical terms, but it is social judgments they are rendering. To say that a man suffers from manic-depressive psychosis is simply to say that he is more agitated or more depressed than the decision maker thinks he should be. You or I could make a similar social decision based on behavior we deem abnormal.

The problem of ambiguity pervades not only the subjective area of behavior evaluation, but also the obstensibly objective realm of the psychiatric terms themselves. Such terms are very flexible and often overlap with nonpsychiatric terms. For example, if Mr. Smith drinks a lot and drifts from job to job, making few friends along the way, he might be called a schizophrenic. Another doctor, less enamored of specialized vocabulary, might say Mr. Smith is an alcoholic. A third might simply say he is an unhappy and unsuccessful man. All three judgments share a common nonmedical point of view: frequent drinking is bad; steady jobs and constant friends are good. Does the psychiatric term help us to understand Mr. Smith any better than the other two? Does it help us decide what we should do for or to him? Obviously not. And yet Mr. Smith's liberty may depend on which term is used. If his ex-wife says he is a bum, he will remain free. If she hires a psychiatrist, who says Mr. Smith is schizophrenic, he might be committed against his will to a mental hospital.

Furthermore, the more ominous psychiatric terms, such as schizophrenia, seem to be applied to white people much less often than to blacks. In 1969, for example, nineteen out of every one hundred white males admitted to state and county mental hospitals were diagnosed as schizophrenic. In the same period, the same hospitals showed a diagnosis of schizophrenia for thirty-six of every hundred black male admissions—nearly twice as many. Since there is no evidence that the condition called schizophrenia occurs more often among blacks than among whites, it seems fair to conclude that behavior labeled schizophrenic in a black man is given a less pejorative name when the patient happens to be white. Perhaps that is why, as the same report showed, nearly forty of every hundred white male admissions were diagnosed as alcoholic, a somewhat more respectable term, compared with thirty out of a hundred black male admissions. There is no evidence that alcoholism occurs more often among whites than among blacks.

The diagnostic differences hold true for women as well, though with different percentages. Out of every one hundred white females admitted to state and county mental hospitals in 1969, thirty-three were diagnosed as schizophrenic and ten as alcoholic. For black female admissions, 52 per cent were diagnosed as schizophrenic and only 3 per cent as alcoholic. These figures suggest, although they do not prove, that psychiatric judgments are racist. Dozens of other studies have concluded that diagnostic decisions, which psychiatrists like to think of as scientific and impartial, are in fact heavily influenced by the race of the prospective patient.

Whatever else these figures and studies show, it is undeniable that the nonwhite rate of admission to state and county mental hospitals is about one and a half times the white rate. In certain age categories, it is even higher. In 1969, out of every 100,000 whites aged twenty-five to thirty-four, 232 were admitted to such hospitals. Out of every 100,000 nonwhites of the same ages, 553 were admitted. That is nearly two and a half times the white admission rate. Similarly, the nonwhite admission rate for persons aged thirty-five to forty-four was more than twice the white rate —632 per 100,000, compared with 308 per 100,000.

But there is no evidence that mental illness occurs less frequently among whites than among nonwhites. Why, then, does a mentally ill white man stand so much better chance of staying out of a mental hospital than does a mentally ill black man or Puerto Rican? Money accounts for much of the difference. A high percentage of blacks and Puerto Ricans in the United States are poor, and poor people cannot afford private psychiatrists, or some of the other alternatives to hospitalization. Even when a free outpatient clinic is available to him, the poor man cannot easily take a day off from work to go there.

And there are more subtle explanations. Call it racism, as I do, or whatever you choose, but it is true that psychiatrists are more careful about stigmatizing persons from their own socioeconomic group than about stigmatizing those whose education and prospects for the future seem, to them, inferior to their own. After all, what does it matter that a history of hospitalization makes it difficult to get into graduate school? Black people don't go to graduate school anyway. It would be too upsetting to the life style of a suburbanite to remove him from his comfortable ranch-style home and put him in a mental hospital. But wouldn't another man be better off in a mental hospital than some rat-infested tenement in East Harlem?

The dimensions of the problem are equally staggering. In 1967, almost 3 million Americans were treated in psychiatric facilities.

More than 800,000 were treated in state and county mental hospitals, 106,000 in private mental hospitals, and 579,000 in the psychiatric wards of general hospitals like Bellevue. Another 1,400,000 were treated in outpatient psychiatric clinics. In the twenty years between 1946 and 1966, the total number of psychiatric facilities in the United States rose from 1,000 to 4,000, and new ones are being built every day.

Instead of constructing more mental hospitals, we would be wiser to build nursing homes, cottage retreats, and similar facilities for senior citizens. If we did, we could cut the mental hospital population drastically. Half the patients in New York State mental hospitals are over sixty; similar rates prevail in other states. In 1966, there were 135,000 resident patients sixty-five or older in this country's state and county mental hospitals. Very few of them needed, or were receiving, psychiatric care; they were simply old and helpless. But instead of providing attractive geriatric facilities, as is done in Scandinavia, we crowd them into the back wards of mental hospitals.

An enormous amount of tax money is consumed in building and operating mental hospitals. In the fiscal year 1970–71, New York State spent almost $600 million for its public mental hospitals and schools for the retarded; the amount was far from adequate. Yet it is not only more money that is needed but also a more sensible allocation of what we have. New York spends about $18 per day for each state hospital patient; Iowa spends about $50 (the national average is about $15). In the long run, however, the taxpayers in Iowa spend a lot less per patient than do the taxpayers in New York. With its higher expenditure, Iowa, unlike New York, is able to hire enough psychiatrists, psychologists, social workers, nurses, and paraprofessionals to give each patient an active treatment program. Consequently, the average period of hospitalization in Iowa is fifteen days, compared to the New York average of sixty days. Fifteen days at $50 per day ($750) is much cheaper than sixty days at $18 per day

($1,080). It would be cheaper still to shut down mental hospitals entirely and treat all patients in the community.

California has come close to doing that. New York, with a population of nearly 19 million, has a state hospital population of about 55,000. California, with a population of nearly 20 million, has a state hospital population of only 11,500, and that number is rapidly declining. To be sure, there are just as many mentally ill people in California as in New York; but in California they do not wind up in hospitals. A new California law limits involuntary hospitalization largely to persons who have committed dangerous acts and are demonstrably dangerous to themselves or to others. Everyone else is treated in the community. Also, by placing presumptive time limits on involuntary hospitalization (fourteen days for persons who are suicidal, and ninety days for those who are homicidal or assaultive), the law ensures that even the so-called dangerous patients will be rapidly returned to the community. In fact, within thirteen days of admission, 95 per cent of all supposedly suicidal patients and 98 per cent of all supposedly dangerous-to-others patients are discharged.

Although the average period of hospitalization is much shorter under the new California law (13 days) than under the old (180 days), the rehospitalization rate is now *lower*, as is the incidence of suicide or antisocial behavior by discharged patients.

California's new law is far from perfect. But it has shown that most people can be treated in the community, and that the few who must be hospitalized can be quickly returned to the community with no adverse consequences.

Other states could duplicate the California experience simply by tightening up their commitment standards and procedures, thus restricting hospital intake. The money no longer needed for huge hospitals could be used to build community-based outpatient facilities.

Of course, stringent commitment standards will not reduce hospital populations if, as is common, they are routinely ignored.

The District of Columbia's commitment standards are more stringent than most ("imminent danger to self or others"), but the District still has the highest rate of hospitalization in the United States—an average of 629 per 100,000 population, according to 1966 figures. (The national average is 238 residents per 100,000 population.) There are two reasons for this unenviable record. The first is that prospective patients are often indiscriminately labeled dangerous. The second reason is more curious. Each year thousands of persons travel to the capital to petition the government for redress of grievances. If, in the opinion of a guard or official, the grievance is imagined, the petitioner, I am told, will be labeled a "White House Crazy" and transported to St. Elizabeth's Hospital.

On the other hand, loose commitment criteria almost guarantee a high rate of hospitalization. New York, which has the loosest criteria in the nation, ranks second only to the District of Columbia in rate of hospitalization (467 residents per 100,000 population). Lest it be thought that "urban stress" explains New York's high rate, note that New Hampshire ranks third. Iowa, which has more doctors per patient than any other state (one for every twenty-four), is able to give more intensive treatment. Not surprisingly, it ranks forty-ninth in the number of mental patients per 100,000 population.

Tightening commitment criteria and placing absolute or presumptive limits on the length of involuntary hospitalization would do much to transform mental hospitals from custodial warehouses to treatment facilities. But even if the system is improved, it will still permit the involuntary incarceration of an individual who has committed no crime. Eventually, we must question the legitimacy of involuntary hospitalization. When we do, we may be surprised how frail its justifications are.

Essentially, there are only two. The first is that in the absence of involuntary hospitalization, the prospective patient would be dangerous to himself or to others. The second is that even if he would not be dangerous, he is mentally ill and needs treatment. Neither justification bears scrutiny.

The first, or "danger," justification reflects a commonly held stereotype of the mentally ill that is simply contrary to fact. Hardly a week goes by that we do not read a newspaper story headlined FORMER MENTAL PATIENT STABS WIFE, or something of the sort. And we remember those headlines. We do not remember, because it is never reported, that each week thousands of former mental patients go about their business without harming or frightening anyone.

The evidence is overwhelming that mental patients and former mental patients are, as a class, less dangerous than the "average" citizen. Witness the New York study showing that over a five-year period the arrest rate for 5,000 former patients, all adult males, was less than one-twelfth the rate for the community at large; the rate for serious crimes was even lower. Those former patients who did brush against the law usually were guilty of no more than loitering, vagrancy, or public intoxication. Other studies of patients and prospective patients have reached the same conclusion: mental illness does not cause dangerous behavior; it inhibits dangerous behavior. Mental patients may plot and scheme, they may threaten injury to themselves or others, but rarely do they follow through. The most common characteristic of mental patients is an inability to organize their lives and assert themselves. And that characteristic makes them *less* dangerous than people who are more aggressive and, hence, more "normal."

True, some mental patients are dangerous—though it is more likely to be in spite of their mental condition than because of it. So we are left with the legitimate question of what to do with persons we believe to be both mentally ill and dangerous.

The problem is one of prediction. We can never be certain that a person will commit a dangerous act. To return to the earlier comparison with criminal law, this uncertainty is why our criminal laws protect the liberty of the individual until after he has committed the criminal act—or, at the least, until after he has committed an overt act that is just short of the crime itself and makes the crime imminent. We do not wait until the gunman holds up the bank before arresting him, but we do wait until he enters the bank gun in hand. After all, at the last moment he might change his mind, or lose his nerve, and continue down the block.

Consider the paradox. Whatever his past, we never put a man in jail because of something he *might* do in the future. If he has not actually committed a dangerous or criminal act, we let him alone, no matter how "sure" we may be that he will do something wrong in the future. Yet we are not at all reluctant to put the same man in a mental hospital. The added ingredient "mental illness" somehow justifies incarceration. We condemn preventive detention of the sane but welcome preventive detention of the insane. But is the victim any happier for learning that his assailant, though dangerous, was sane and thus left at liberty? If we really wanted to prevent future dangerous behavior, we would incarcerate everyone considered dangerous, sane or not.

Why, then, do we single out the mentally ill for preventive detention? The answer is complex. We do so, in part, for historical reasons—it has always been done that way—and in part for sociological reasons—mental patients are considered second-class citizens whose rights need not be respected as strenuously as the rights of the sane. Furthermore, our reasons are often dishonest; we do not really think they are dangerous, but we want them put away and are therefore willing to label them dangerous. Often, we are not aware of our dishonesty, and may have convinced ourselves that they are dangerous—at least to themselves —in order to lessen whatever guilt we feel about hospitalizing them.

But the main reasons we single out the mentally ill for preventive detention stem from ignorance and from overconfidence.

We are certain that the mentally ill are more dangerous than the sane, and we are equally certain that we can predict future dangerous behavior more accurately with the mentally ill than with the sane.

We have already seen that the so-called mentally ill, as a class, are not more dangerous than the sane. Accordingly, even if psychiatrists could single out the individuals who were in some objective sense mentally ill—and they cannot—they would have to go further and determine which of those diagnosed as mentally ill were also dangerous. They cannot do that, either. There is absolutely nothing in the education, training, or experience of psychiatrists to enable them to predict dangerous behavior. In fact, psychiatrists are less accurate predictors of dangerous behavior than are policemen.

In a well-known New York study, psychiatrists predicted that 989 persons were so dangerous that they could not be kept even in civil mental hospitals, but would have to be kept in maximum security hospitals run by the Department of Corrections. Then, because of a United States Supreme Court decision, those persons were transferred to civil hospitals. After a year, the Department of Mental Hygiene reported that one-fifth of them had been discharged to the community, and over half had agreed to remain as voluntary patients. During the year, only 7 of the 989 committed or threatened any act that was sufficiently dangerous to require retransfer to the maximum security hospital. Seven correct predictions out of almost a thousand is not a very impressive record.

Other studies, and there are many, have reached the same conclusion: psychiatrists simply cannot predict dangerous behavior. They are wrong more often than they are right. And they always err by overpredicting dangerous behavior.

There are also philosophical and practical objections to the "need-for-treatment" justification, which authorizes the involuntary hospitalization of nondangerous persons on the ground that it will be good for them.

The essential premise of liberty is that people can do whatever they want—including things that are bad for them—so long as they do not injure others. We permit people to smoke, though we know smoking shortens lives. We permitted Justice Robert Jackson to resume his seat on the United States Supreme Court after a heart attack, though his doctors had told him, correctly, that the work load would cause a fatal attack within a year. We allow persons to give away their fortunes, destituting themselves for a cause. Every day, each of us does something that another would criticize, or fails to do something that another would urge. That is what liberty means.

Consider the patient in a general hospital with a physical, rather than a mental, disease. He has the legal right to refuse surgery, though it may save his life. We might think he has made a wrong or irrational decision, but he is permitted to make it. Transfer the same patient down the corridor to the psychiatric wing of the hospital, and he will no longer be permitted to make the decisions that affect his life.

Why is this so? Why is it that persons can do whatever they want with their lives until the moment someone else says they are mentally ill? Why is it that mental patients are stripped of rights that the general patient, and everyone else, can take for granted? It is because we accept without question the assumption that the mental patient, if sane, would choose for himself exactly what the doctors say he should choose.

There are many problems with that assumption. The first is that it is self-fulfilling. It can never be proved wrong because disagreement with the doctor is itself considered evidence of insanity.

We have seen that, contrary to popular assumption, a diagnosis of mental illness tells us nothing about whether the individual is dangerous. Similarly, a diagnosis of mental illness tells us nothing about his capacity to make rational decisions (even accepting the doctor's definition of rational).* Some mental patients can make what doctors would consider rational decisions, and some cannot. In New York state hospitals, for example, there are thousands of voluntary patients. The doctors would say that although those persons are mentally ill, they have nevertheless made a rational choice—to hospitalize themselves for treatment. In other words, mental illness of itself does not render a person incapable of making rational decisions.

On the philosophical level, therefore, a diagnosis of mental illness does not end the inquiry. It is still necessary, in each case, to determine whether the prospective patient's decision to resist hospitalization is rational or not. At this point, we confront insuperable difficulties.

Even if we assume that a hospitalized patient will receive treatment that will improve his mental condition, we must also take into consideration the adverse consequences of hospitalization. Is it rational to enter a mental hospital when you know that upon discharge you will have lost your apartment and your job, and will have a hard time finding others? Hospitalization creates disabilities of its own, and it costs a lot of money, which the patient, if able, must pay.

Thus, there would be good reasons for avoiding hospitalization even if it made you better. And in fact it is likely to make you worse.

It is worth repeating that hospitalization is itself antitherapeutic. Psychiatrists have a word for it—institutionalization. It is hard to imagine a more depressing environment than the sullen corridors and empty hours of a state mental hospital. A man signs himself into a hospital because he fears that he and his life

* Sample ballots given to all the patients at Bronx State Hospital in New York City showed that their votes for president, governor, and mayor were not statistically different from the votes of the citizens in the communities from which they had been admitted.

have no importance. Once there, his fears are confirmed. Rarely will a doctor stop to speak with him; and when he does, it is only to ask his name, whether he is working, and if he knows the day and date. The doctor asks nothing at all about his past, his hopes, his life—there is no time for that. The patient will wear the same clothes as the other patients, eat the same food, receive the same medication, watch the same TV shows, and fall asleep in a long room filled with fifty or sixty metal beds exactly alike.

The hard fact is that mental hospitals do not treat; they degrade. Perhaps 5 per cent of the patients are in some sort of treatment program; for the rest there is nothing. In 1958, Dr. Harry Solomon, who was then president of the American Psychiatric Association, declared that our public mental hospitals were bankrupt beyond repair. They still are.

Mental hospitals are not what they claim to be, and exposing institutional psychiatry for what it is is a necessary step toward reform. But, unfortunately, coercive psychiatry has found a comfortable niche in society. How would we tame our rebellious young, or rid ourselves of doddering parents, or clear the streets of the offensive poor, without it? Although a frontal attack on the concept of involuntary hospitalization will likely have little impact, some hope may lie in legal attack. So much is wrong with involuntary hospitalization that a reasonable tightening up of commitment standards and a modest extension of patients' rights would cripple the enterprise beyond recovery.

For example, limiting the application of the "danger" standard to persons who have recently committed or threatened substantial physical injury to self or to others would mean that all but a handful of those now hospitalized as dangerous would have to be released. Similarly, requiring hospitals to show that they provide something more than the same food, clothing, shelter, and structured environment one finds in a prison would force the discharge of most patients now hospitalized because they "are in need of care and treatment." Abolishing patient labor, or requiring hospitals to pay fair value for that labor, would shut down the hospitals in several states.

The most effective short-range reform, however, would be to require the mandatory assignment of counsel and a mandatory judicial hearing (unless affirmatively waived by the patient after consultation with the counsel), either before or promptly after hospitalization. That does not sound like much. Everyone, after all, should have the right to a lawyer before he is stripped of his liberty, labeled mad, and bussed away, perhaps for life, to a mental hospital. But consider the consequences.

There are, in the United States, about 500,000 practicing lawyers. Each year, almost 2 million Americans wind up, for some period of time, as patients in a public mental hospital. At present, most lawyers retire without ever having represented a mental patient. If the courts would diligently assign counsel to represent each patient, every lawyer in this country would have to represent at least four patients each year. Before long, the lawyers, either shocked by the conditions they encountered or annoyed at the amount of time spent on nonpaying cases, would change the system.

If the state paid the lawyers for their time—say $250 per case— the nationwide bill would amount to $500 million per year. And if full-scale judicial hearings were the norm rather than the exception, there would not be nearly enough judges to handle the load.

Bellevue, for example, averages 10,000 to 15,000 involuntary admissions each year, but only about 500 judicial hearings. Suppose half of the patients admitted received hearings. Where would we get the judges to hear them, or the courtrooms to hear them in?

What does all this mean? It means that the mental hospital system depends for its existence on the premise that mental patients are second-class citizens entitled to fewer protections than persons accused of crime. Under the guise of not treating patients like criminals, the system has treated patients *worse* than criminals.

It is time to change that. The goal should be nothing less than the abolition of involuntary hospitalization. That will not come soon, but it will come. (England, for example, plans to shut down all its large public mental hospitals within twenty years.) Short of that, there is still much we could do. We could insist that patients in mental hospitals be given the same rights and privileges as patients in general hospitals. We could demand that legislators spend our tax dollars for community-based outpatient treatment facilities, rather than for custodial warehouses.

Of course, we could have done these things last year or the year before. But no one bothered.